AF797178

Our Daughter's Heart

Our Daughter's Heart

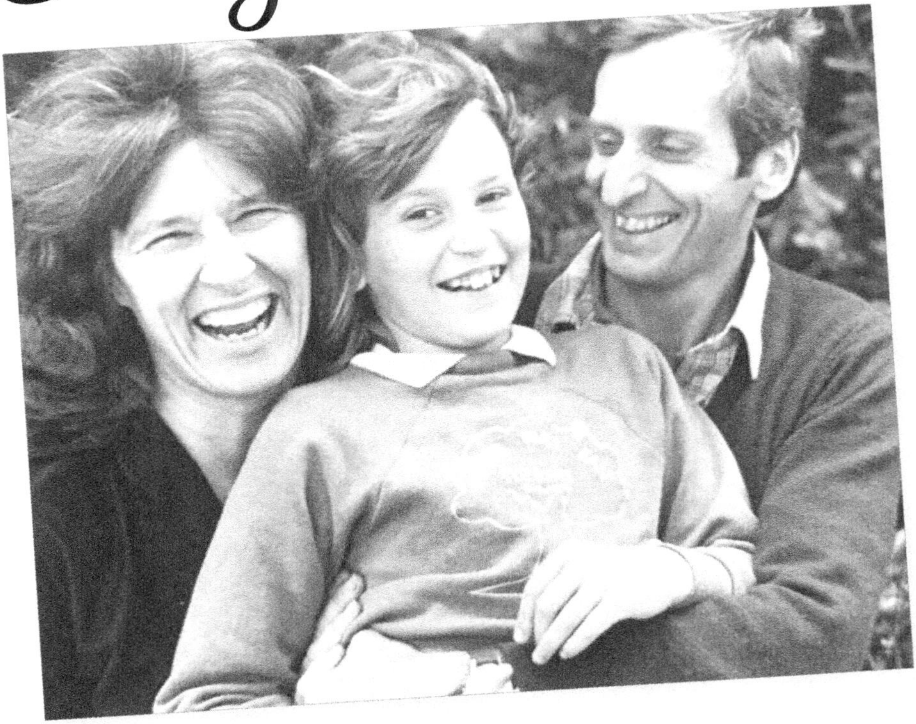

Dorothy Stoneman

Copyright © 2021 by Dorothy Stoneman.

ISBN 978-1-7368556-0-7

All rights reserved.

CONTENTS

PREFACE vii
PROLOGUE 1
INTRODUCTION 5
1. Some Background 9
2. Sierra Meets Dr. Doyle 15
3. Unexpected Lessons 21
4. Sierra Learns of the Coming Operation 31
5. We Inform and Confuse Ourselves 35
6. Sierra Gets Ahead of Us 51
7. The Letter 65
8. Mistakes 89
9. Sierra Decides 93
10. Final Preparations 99
11. The Roller Coaster 117
12. The Crisis 133
13. The Collapse 145
14. The Aftermath 155
PHOTO ALBUM 161
15. Try Again 173
16. The Recovery Room 181
17. The Intensive Care Unit 185
18. Life . . . and Death . . . Goes On 189
19. Thirteen Years Later 191
EPILOGUE: REFLECTIONS FROM SIERRA, 39 YEARS LATER 195

PREFACE

When a family faces a major medical crisis, a complex set of feelings, decisions, and relationships are set into motion. When the crisis involves a young child, it is especially laden with emotion. It tests each thread of the family fabric—the systems of belief and faith, the community to which the family belongs, the childrearing theories that are consciously or unconsciously guiding the parents, and the financial structure that holds the family up. The family's response draws on all its resources and all its conditioning, and is profoundly influenced by the religious, educational, cultural, and class backgrounds of the parents.

When my husband and I discovered that our little daughter would need major heart surgery, we entered new territory. She was nine months old when we learned that she would need major surgery at age four. Figuring out how to handle our own and our daughter's feelings, while interacting with a medical establishment of which we had minimal knowledge and over which we had even less influence, took concentration. The situation seemed fraught with dangers, and there was precious little guidance available to help us handle it wisely. Our conditioning as middle-class professionals established the basic assumption that we had a right and an obligation to understand and influence our experience. But beyond that, we hadn't the foggiest notion of what to do.

To help keep my perspective and my emotional balance, I kept a very thorough diary. I hoped that a record of how we handled it could turn out to be useful for other parents facing similar ordeals.

Despite the availability of the best imaginable medical care, it was indeed an ordeal, and one that hovered over our lives for years in advance and lasted for months in the crunch.

Our intent was to handle it in such a way that our child would physically survive the operation, that the emotional experience for her would be reassuring rather than traumatic, and that our family would be strengthened rather than strained. Fortunately, we were successful in all three respects, but not without lots of soul-searching and research, some drama, and some setbacks.

I hope the following account of our experience will be helpful to other parents. Maintaining the diary was certainly helpful to me in maintaining my balance during the events.

Dorothy Stoneman, September 2020

PROLOGUE

by John Bell

Husband and Partner of Dorothy Stoneman
& Father of Sierra Stoneman–Bell.

It's May 1981. I'm alone in the parents' lounge at New York University Medical Center. Sierra, our precious five-year-old daughter, is downstairs in the operating room receiving heart surgery to correct a coarctation of her aorta. Without this surgery she would likely die by the time she is twenty, because the narrowing of her aorta constricts the blood flow to the lower half of her body. We've known about this since she was nine months old, but her heart had to grow more to allow for a greater chance of successful surgery. Today's the day.

My wife, Dorothy, and two friends, Lisel Burns and Tom Roderick, have been with me during this excruciating wait. They just stepped out for few minutes. As a family, we prepared for years for this day. But now I'm scared. In the quiet of the room, by myself, I start to pray. I was raised Catholic but have not been practicing for decades. When I was a boy, I felt an intimate closeness to Jesus, so, in this moment of crisis, I find myself reflexively praying to Jesus and to God to bring Sierra safely through the operation. I am crying and shaking with fear. Suddenly I am struck by a new thought: Life is asking something deeper of me. At this moment,

Sierra's life is in the hands of the surgeon and the medical staff. I am powerless. Life is asking me to be okay with whatever happens, even if she dies on the operating table. Life is telling me that I am not in control, that things don't always work out the way I want, that I have to surrender to the unfathomable mystery of life. This realization released a huge new vat of tears, of relief, of worry. A kind of peace spread over me. It was okay.

That was forty years ago. Sierra survived beautifully, flourished in all directions, and now has her own son who, at the time of this writing, is about the same age she was at the time of her heart surgery. Dorothy took notes during the whole process of our family's multiyear preparation and unpredictable experiences leading up to the surgery. This book tells that full and dramatic story. When she wrote the first draft a few years after the surgery, publishers said that our parenting ways were too unusual and they declined to publish our story. So it languished for decades. But now, as we sit in the midst of the 2020 COVID-19 pandemic, the issues of life and death are again front and center. So we think the timelessness of this story is ripe for sharing.

Hundreds of thousands of parents worldwide face the daunting and heartbreaking prospect of major surgery for their child, and living through those scary hours of entrusting their child to strangers in the operating room. Whether or not they have a moment of spiritual opening like I did, the preparation, the flow of medical information and procedures, the range of emotions, and the feelings of worry or uncertainty or powerlessness or fear or confusion are intense for all parents in this situation. For most parents, this is new territory for which they are unprepared. Our way of handling Sierra's preparation for the surgery grow out of our own backgrounds and beliefs, and may seem somewhat unconventional to many, but we hope some of the underlying principles and approaches are helpful.

By reading this book, besides enjoying a dramatic and well-told story, you will learn about how we did our best to respect the intelligence of our daughter at every step and included her in many decisions; how we learned to navigate the medical system and be advocates for Sierra, even bucking the doctors occasionally when we felt it was necessary; how we used stories, humor, and role playing with her over and over again on every aspect of the doctors' visits, the hospitalizations, the repetitive testing and shots, the surgery itself and recovery; how we encouraged Sierra to ask her questions and feel her feelings at every step, and welcomed her tears or anger or need for comforting or appropriate information; how we created a support system for ourselves to release our own emotions, given the roller coaster nature of the process that lasted several years.

In our preparation, we heard stories and read helpful books about other parents' and children's experiences preparing for major childhood surgery. We think this book adds some unique and unconventional perspectives. May it be a reassuring friend for parents facing the challenge.

John Bell, September 2020

INTRODUCTION

January 1980

Sierra is a lovely, joyous, strong-minded child of four years and three quarters. She has the qualities of a beloved only child. She is very articulate and confident, very kind and trusting. She believes she is very lucky because she has friends who give her Valentine's Day presents. She thinks people should always keep their promises, never hurt each other's feelings, never flush the toilet or let the faucet drip when there's a water shortage, and always care for lonely animals by bringing them in (to our house) off the streets of New York. She is kind to her friends, and is frequently heard saying, "In our family you're allowed to cry, because my parents tell people not to say mean things to crying children."

Sierra is also stubborn, like an Amazon child. She wears Wonder Woman underwear. If she wants a piece of candy, she'll mount a tantrum out on Broadway that will last half an hour and gather a small crowd of onlookers who try to decide whether this child needs a good spanking or her mother needs to be taken in on child-abuse charges. Her screams are unrestrained. At the very top of her formidable lungs she will scream, "DON'T DO THAT TO ME, NOOOO! MOMMY! DON'T TREAT ME LIKE THIS!! DON'T! PLEASE DON'T! STOP!" She'll fly at me in a rage, trying to hurt me with her little fists, because sometimes I don't give her what she wants when she wants it.

Sierra has a congenital heart defect that could cause her to die in her early twenties from brain hemorrhaging if the defect is not corrected by major surgery in her childhood. We've known of this possibility since she was a perfect nine-month-old baby.

I remember so vividly the evening after our pediatrician, Rodney Hite, first told us about the defect. Sierra and I were home alone together. I was sitting in the big brown stuffed chair in the corner, by the window, watching her crawl intently around our bedroom, exploring all the bureau drawers. I called my friend Tony Ward and wept the bad news into the telephone as I watched her. I felt like I was in another world. I couldn't believe there was anything wrong with her heart. Nobody in my family had ever been sick. How could Sierra have a serious heart defect requiring surgery? She had no symptoms. She was perfect. What could be wrong inside that healthy little body?

But it was true. The pediatrician had found a heart murmur, and had found no pulse in the lower half of her body. He sent us to a cardiologist, who said Sierra probably had a coarctation of the aorta, a narrowing in the major artery that takes all the blood from the heart. This narrowing would give her extremely high blood pressure as the heart worked to get the blood through it, and that could easily kill her in her early twenties from hemorrhaging in the brain.

But then we put it out of our minds because Rodney told us he'd "watch it clinically, do no intrusive tests, and see what developed." After a year or so, he didn't hear the murmur. So we relaxed, until the day when a preoccupied look came over his face as he put his stethoscope over and over again to all the spots on her back. Over and over again he listened, looking faraway, concentrating. Then he folded up his stethoscope, slowly.

He was so agitated, I knew it was serious. Then he said:

> She still has the murmur. It sounds like coarctation, which does require surgery. We'll go through all the necessary tests . . . oh, I'm sorry. I knew when I became a pediatrician that a certain statistical percentage of my patients would come up with serious problems, but I always hate it when it happens. I know a few will have heart problems, and a few will have leukemia, and a few will have other diseases, but always I hate it when it happens.

You hate it, I thought. *Back off. You're not helping me by telling me how upset you are. And these things shouldn't be said in front of Sierra. She might get alarmed.* So I signaled that we shouldn't pursue it, and I'd call him later.

When I called him later, he said, at the end of our conversation, "Just remember that I love Sierra and you and John, and I'll be right there with you through the whole ordeal." I hung up with a catch in my throat and very mixed feelings. I was very grateful to him for really caring, but I was very scared by how seriously he was taking this. I guessed we were in for a real, full, life crisis.

I picked the phone back up and called the cardiologist for an appointment. When I told the secretary that my daughter probably had a coarctation, she said, "Oh, I'm so sorry to hear that. Let me connect you with the doctor right away." My fear was mounting rapidly. If the people working for the heart specialist were so sorry, we must be in for some very rough times. We got our first reassurance when we visited Dr. Eugenie Doyle, the cardiologist. She confirmed that it was a coarctation and would require surgery between ages four and five. But she said the operation was not so bad. Only two percent die from it. "If you must have a serious problem," she said, "this is the best serious problem to have."

We believed her. Since we had never had a serious problem before, we figured that maybe we did have to have one someday, and this was it.

CHAPTER ONE

Some Background

(written in 1984)

JOHN BELL AND I met in 1968 in New York City, where we both taught public school. We were married in 1974, and gave birth to Sierra in 1976. John grew up on the West Coast, I on the East.

John is a thin, blonde, blue-eyed, and craggy-faced man who grew up within sight of Mount Rainier. He was a devoted altar boy in the Catholic Church. He loves music, mountains, and meditation. He has a gift for being a child therapist, which expressed itself professionally through his being a teacher of young children, and personally by his being the wonderfully kind and playful father most of us dreamed of and few of us ever had.

He is an extremely thoughtful and caring person, occasionally suffering from overcontrol of his feelings and a resulting sense of loneliness. He always does the right thing whether he feels like it or not, so he sometimes loses track of how he feels. People around him feel one hundred percent safe and trusting because John would never hurt a soul. He will always be strongly and thoughtfully human.

I am an energetic, brown-haired activist, half Russian Jew and half German Protestant, raised in the suburbs of Boston as a Unitarian Girl Scout. I have been a teacher and community organizer from the day I joined the civil rights movement in 1964, and probably well before that, if I think of the babysitting I did as a child and the social organizing I did as a teenager. I love children and dogs and back-packing, and I hate for people to be mistreated. I suffer from feeling that nothing I do is enough, and that everything wrong is my responsibility. I sometimes wake up at night with obsessive worries, which John then wakes up to dispel with various kinds of reassurances so I can go back to sleep.

Sierra, John, and I live together in New York City, in Central Harlem, in a brownstone shared with other tenants. We live on a friendly, tree-lined block in which neighbors keep an eye out for each other, and crime is minimal because the residents are organized to keep it off the block. There are four or five families near us with small children, so, on a nice day, the children go from house to house, running in and out almost as they would in the suburbs. Nonetheless, it would be nice to have a yard in front of the house instead of pavement.

We have both been teachers in Harlem since the mid-sixties, and have lived on 137th Street between Adam Clayton Powell Boulevard (Seventh Avenue) and Frederick Douglas Boulevard (Eighth Avenue), since 1970. In 1978 I founded the Youth Action Program in East Harlem to engage teenagers in community improvement projects of their own design. I had been struck when I first came to Harlem in 1964 at how hard it would be to raise a teenager in a context with so many street temptations and so few organized opportunities for work, education, recreation, and political activity. When a young man who had been one of my favorite second-grade students years earlier died as a young teenager by falling, or being pushed, off a roof, I decided to do my part in changing the conditions of life for teenagers. The Youth Action Program was the result. By 1980 it was a thriving and demanding network of youth-run community improvement projects that had gained national attention for its unusual encouragement of young people to be leaders and decision-makers. John and I were both giving it the bulk of our time and emotional energy. Nonetheless, from the moment we learned that surgery for Sierra would be necessary, we began, slowly, to prepare. We assumed that Sierra would need very gradual and unthreatening information, given steadily over a period of time, to prepare her for what loomed ahead as a terrifying and life-threatening experience.

We also assumed that we ourselves would need lots of information and lots of emotional support in order to rid ourselves of the dread, so we could handle it wisely. We wanted our approach to give Sierra confidence that everything would be okay.

Throughout all the preparations, which began in 1978 and ended with the operation itself in 1981, both strands coexisted: deep and irrational dread, causing John and me to imagine her body scarred, her ribs broken, her body paralyzed, her brain damaged, her life destroyed, her precious self dead as a result of failed surgery; and at the same time going ahead with gentle, careful, thorough and thoughtful preparations to enable all of us to handle this family crisis gracefully. We knew it would need our attention, and if we turned our attention to handling it right, it could, if all went well, strengthen our family and our daughter. Poorly handled, we thought it could explode us into distress.

We knew our hurdles would be both general ones—ones that any family facing crisis would have to handle—and very unique ones, rooted in our peculiar individual forms of anxiety and worry.

One general hurdle was that of time and money. Both of us work, and between us we earn $23,000 a year. Fortunately, the Youth Action Program gives us full health coverage. We also work extremely hard, leaving very little time. It was unclear how we could break away enough time to attend to Sierra's special needs.

Another general hurdle was deciding how we would prepare Sierra emotionally and intellectually. It is our strong conviction that children need to be fully informed, consulted, and included in family experiences. They need to be given as much information as possible and encouraged to think about sophisticated things. They need their intelligence respected, their feelings heard, and their ability to make decisions honored.

A unique hurdle peculiar to my own psyche was my tendency to feel guilty. Not only did I dread that something awful would happen, but I knew that I would find a way to blame myself permanently for any tragedy, if I believed I had in any way shirked the preparations. I made up my mind to go all the way with this. No matter what happened, I had to know that I had given it my best.

I decided that I would arrange to take a two-month leave of absence from work, and that I would also start spending more time with Sierra well in advance of the operation. Since I am always busy, Sierra misses me a lot. I definitely did not want her to conclude that going to the hospital was the most reliable way to get Mommy's attention.

Of these hurdles, the most interesting one was determining how we would prepare Sierra. How and when would we tell her? How much would we tell her? How would we make sure she wouldn't have a terrible, traumatic experience that would permanently affect her trust in the world and in us?

CHAPTER TWO

Sierra Meets Dr. Doyle

THE CENTRAL FIGURE IN our medical lives became Dr. Eugenie Doyle, the supremely competent cardiologist who led us through the maze of information, fear, and crisis between 1979 and 1981.

We had found her pretty much by accident. No big search for the best cardiologist. Once when Rodney was out of town, Sierra had an ear infection requiring attention, so we took her to another pediatrician. When this doctor listened to her heart, he matter-of-factly said, "She has a heart murmur. It's not a benign one. She will probably need surgery. Here's the name of a very good cardiologist at New York University Medical Center." When we reported this interaction to Rodney, he agreed that Dr. Doyle was excellent. He referred us formally to her. It turned out that Dr. Doyle, the head of the Pediatric Cardiology Department at New York University Medical Center, was widely respected in her field. She was considered "an institution" by the staff and trainees at the hospital. We were very lucky.

Sierra was just three years old in the spring of 1979 when we scheduled her to see Dr. Doyle for the first time. This appointment posed the first challenge regarding what to tell Sierra, how much to tell her, and when to tell her. She needed to know why she was going to see a new doctor.

Her experience with doctors in the past had been emotion-ridden. When she was eighteen months old, due to a painful throat culture that he had taken when she had a viciously swollen throat, Sierra had become terrified of Rodney. She was so terrified that when he walked into the room a look of extreme fear gripped her and she began screaming.

It had taken six months to free her of that terror. During that time we had refused to let him touch her, and had insisted that he could only listen to her heart, look in her ears, and give her a shot when she had sufficient verbal comprehension to understand why these things were necessary, and until she gave her permission.

We used the book *Curious George Goes to the Hospital* as a way for Sierra to face her feelings; at her request, we read it dozens of times and talked about every detail of it over and over. After this, we made friendly visits to the doctor in his office when she was perfectly healthy and needed no treatment. Finally, at age two, Sierra announced that Rodney was her friend and gave him permission to give her a shot.

We had, in this way, already put a lot of work into Sierra's relationship with doctors. We were prepared to handle this new relationship with Dr. Doyle pretty tenderly.

We asked Dr. Doyle if Sierra's best friend, Annie Thoms, could come with her to the examination. Dr. Doyle readily agreed. This was important, because Annie had played a key role in helping Sierra get over her fear of Rodney. By coincidence, Rodney was also Annie's pediatrician. Annie and Sierra had several times gone together to his office, and had dramatized shot-giving at the doctor's office many times in their dramatic play. Annie had had a little hernia operation when she was one and a half, so she had ample interest in medical drama. Being six months younger than Annie, Sierra had the greatest admiration for her very knowledgeable friend.

About a week before the scheduled visit, I asked Annie, "Would you like to come with Sierra to meet her new doctor next week?" Annie said, "Yes. But why is Sierra going to meet a new doctor?" Here was my opportunity to explain. With both of them listening avidly, I said, "Sierra has a different sound in her heart. Instead of her heart going *boom-boom, boom-boom, boom-boom,* like most people's hearts, it goes *boom-boom-sshhhh, boom-boom-sshhhh, boom-boom-sshhhh.* We're going to Dr. Doyle so she can find out why. She knows all about hearts."

They both thought this was very funny. *Boom-boom-sshhhh, boom-boom-sshhh*h, said with a lilt, became Sierra's root understanding that something was different about her heart. Why does Sierra's heart go *boom-boom-sshhhh*? That was the question for Dr. Doyle to figure out.

I found that telling Sierra a new thing in the presence of her friends was a very effective way of communicating. It made it all very natural, just a part of conversation. It meant her friends could ask questions, helping Sierra clarify her own questions. It meant Sierra knew there was no big secret or hard thing—she could talk about it with her friends all she wanted.

Out first family trip to Dr. Doyle was delightful. John and I had our hearts in our mouths. For us it was the beginning of a long and scary sequence. But we kept it very light for Sierra and Annie, talking, walking on stone walls, playing in the revolving doors, exploring the medical center.

Dr. Doyle turned out to be an older woman with blonde hair who had a warm, competent, no-nonsense manner. She created a relationship with Sierra in one minute flat by directing a very powerful and calm beacon of attention toward her and expecting her to cooperate while asking questions about what foods Sierra liked and didn't like. Dr. Doyle let Annie squeeze the bulb of the blood pressure gadget, winning both of their hearts.

This was the day Dr. Doyle told us that if we had to have a serious problem, coarctation was the best one to have. Her manner was so forthright and confident, our anxiety drained away. This was to occur over and over again. Every time we saw Dr. Doyle our level of anxiety dropped about fifty percent. It was so obvious we were in good hands.

It was May 1979. Dr. Doyle said Sierra should return to see her the following January, and surgery should occur sometime between age four and age five, between May 1980, and May 1981.

Rodney told us we should not schedule an operation in June because there was a major turnover in interns and residents, meaning that the outgoing staff was overconfident and the incoming staff inexperienced. Better, he said, to schedule surgery some time between September and April. We started aiming for November 1980.

CHAPTER THREE

Unexpected Lessons

On November 15, 1979, Sierra was admitted to Lenox Hill Hospital in the middle of the night as an emergency case. She had intense pain in her abdomen. Appendicitis was suspected.

We were terrified that an emergency operation would have to be performed, which could be complicated due to her high blood pressure. We were concerned that she was about to get a premature exposure to the hospital, making her heart surgery even more traumatic.

But the Lenox Hill experience turned out to be a wonderful piece of Sierra's preparation for the surgery. It was also an important piece of our preparation.

Up until Lenox Hill, I was convinced that Sierra would not be able to handle the needles, the intravenous feeding, the myriad intrusive and annoying incursions of medical procedures in a hospital. She had always been so resistant to these things, and we had always been so incapable of forcing her to submit to them, that I feared the hospital would be a nightmare of coercion by doctors while I stood by trembling. Since I had long ago decided not to abdicate my role as Sierra's protector even when the "attacker" was a doctor, and since I'd never been too good with coercion even when it seemed necessary, I was anxious about how I would handle it. But it turned out that Sierra was able to go through whatever painful experiences we said were necessary with no apparent emotional scars, as long as we remained physically close, as long as we explained everything we knew to her and gave her ample warning, as long as we encouraged her to yell and cry if necessary while the event was taking place, and as long as we did not communicate any great anxieties or fears to her.

In the four days at Lenox Hill, Sierra had three blood tests from her vein, two rectal exams, three chest x-rays, an electrocardiogram, two enemas, at least twenty-seven pokings of her painful stomach, two blood pressure tests, and a day and a half of intravenous feeding after an excruciatingly painful effort by the doctors to find a vein that would work. These things came one after another from a seemingly endless stream of doctors, nurses, and aides.

We had to learn to help her through these things. We had to hold her down, force her to submit, explain to her, listen to her screams and arguments, and still insist it was necessary.

At the same time, we had to figure out and screen out all unnecessary medical procedures and ward off any insensitive medical personnel. There were some of both, despite the basically fine medical care we were getting. Being Sierra's parents in this alien world of pain and medicine was totally demanding and exhausting. It was intensified by our knowledge that this was a minuscule challenge compared to what we would face a year hence.

The hardest part was the intravenous feeding. Sierra was somewhat dehydrated. Since she vomited up even a drop of water, the surgeon said it would be "eminently desirable" to get her on intravenous feeding promptly, both to relieve the dehydration and to prepare for the surgery if it turned out to be necessary. I had a morbid fear of IV, so when the resident doctors came to initiate it, I pulled John aside and said, "Please ask them again if it's really necessary." They said it was and asked that John and I not be in the room during the procedure. John explained that it was important to us and to Sierra that we be there. They unexpectedly yielded.

John, Sierra, myself, and two doctors crowded into a little room on the ward and closed the door. The doctors told Sierra to lie down on her back, but she refused and I moved in, saying, "It'll be easier for all of us if I hold her." Sierra put one arm around me, tight, and held her other arm out to the doctors. I held her tightly, too, with my face away from the needles. The doctors began probing her little hand for a vein. Sierra began screaming, and John left the room as nausea, dizziness, and all the physical symptoms of a short-circuited intelligence flooded him.

Sierra was sobbing and screaming, "Hurry up! Hurry up! Take it out! Take it out. Take it out. Take it out. Take it out! Take it out! Take it out. . ." It seemed interminable. Finally, I looked and saw this red-faced doctor shoving a little needle deeply in and out of Sierra's hand, failing to find a vein.

He was on the second vein when I heard him say, "I guess we've blown this vein, now what shall we do . ." and I saw blood coming in and out of the needle. Suddenly my vision dimmed, my stomach churned, and I saw these doctors as torturers whom it was my parental duty to stop and who might otherwise kill Sierra with their mistakes.

Somehow, I was aware that my feelings were overblown, so I tried reasoning through my dizziness. I forced some reasonable sounding words out of my mouth: "Wouldn't it be better if it's so hard to get the veins, to stop and ask the surgeon if this is really necessary? After all, she might just be constipated, and Dr. Dickinson said it wasn't necessary, just eminently desirable."

I don't remember what exactly they said, but I know it wasn't that they would stop! The next five minutes are a complete blur. I think John was back, recovered. I announced I was about to faint, left the room, returned in a moment determined not to abandon Sierra, but saw John relaxedly back in charge and left again to avoid panicking Sierra with my fainting. I didn't faint—I went to sit on the toilet, cried a minute, prayed a second, and decided to call the expert doctor myself to find out if IV was in fact necessary. Since my brain had short-circuited on lack of knowledge, I decided to get the knowledge.

I put in an emergency call to Rodney, who was our attending pediatrician in the hospital. He explained:

> It is necessary. Sierra is dehydrated. Dr. Pucci said he could smell ketones on her breath. She's acidotic. Her

blood vessels are constricted due to the dehydration; this makes it harder to find the vein. The dehydrating also makes the blood more viscous, increasing her blood pressure. Her pressure is already extremely high due to the constriction in her aorta. Not to begin hydrating her now would mean that if an appendectomy is necessary she would be going into it as an emergency operation rather than a routine one and with her cardiovascular complications it could be dangerous. Furthermore, there is no possible way the doctors can kill Sierra by doing an IV, no matter how bad a mistake they make. They are not going to inject 50cc of air into her veins, and there's no way, ultimately, they can fail to find a vein. If necessary, they will make an incision to get at it. It is not unusual to have to make several tries, especially with a dehydrated child.

I was relieved and persuaded, so I returned to help Sierra get through it. I found her sitting comfortably on John's lap with the needle neatly installed in her hand. After a few minutes of relief, comforting, talking, etc., I went to call my friend Tom Roderick to weep profusely for ten minutes, during which time I remembered a photograph of some torturers in Brazil putting needles into captured guerrillas' arms, from which they were draining all the blood as a method of killing the captives. I suddenly understood my morbid fear of IV.

Fifteen minutes after the IV was inserted, Sierra did move her bowels and begin to recover. But the *drip-drip-drip* of the IV also seemed helpful to her dry little body.

For Sierra to get through each major procedure required firmness on our part that it had to be done, ample explanation in advance about what it was and why it was necessary, and lots of physical closeness during the thing itself. She clung to us tightly during each trauma and yelled at the top of her lungs, but held the affected part of her body still and sometimes yelled intelligent instructions to the doctors. For instance, during her second enema she hollered through her tears that the nurses should count to ten again, as they had the first time, so she would know how long it would be.

For us as parents to get through each procedure required similar conviction that it was necessary, and ample advance warning. It seemed Sierra trusted us to decide what she had to do partly because she noticed that at times we said, "No" to what we knew were unnecessary intrusions. For example, I let her take off the wrist bracelet since she wasn't going to surgery; I insisted on no rectal temperatures since fever was not the main issue; I refused a final blood test the morning she was to leave the hospital, because she was already recovered; I refused a throat culture by the resident doctor because our attending pediatrician had just finished describing all necessary steps for the day and had not included a throat culture. These refusals were not always well taken by the resident doctors. The nurses seemed more flexible, or more willing to yield to parent and patient pressure. But the resident doctors seemed under great pressure in their professional training to succeed, that is, to perform all tests, promptly and professionally.

On the humorous side, one night I was sleeping on the floor under Sierra's bed, because it was more comfortable for my sore back than the parents' lounge chair. I woke up, hearing Sierra crying. I scrambled out from under the bed to find a nurse having pulled off Sierra's pamper preparing to insert a thermometer into her rectum. It was a rude way of awakening Sierra, in my opinion, and I was convinced that sleep, at that point, was the most important thing in her recovery. In my own stupor, I stopped the nurse, who was visibly alarmed by my abrupt appearance from under the bed. She summoned the doctor on duty. He and I argued it out.

"I specifically ordered a rectal temperature," he said. "It's more accurate."

"But the difference won't be more than a half a degree, and her fever is surely no more than 101 degrees, so you can take it under her arm. What will you do differently in her treatment if her fever is 101 and not 100.6 degrees?"

Back and forth, back and forth, until he said, "Well, do you refuse?" and I said, "Yes, I refuse." Only at this point did I realize that I had the legal right to refuse. He whirled on his heels and stalked out, muttering softly.

The next day I had another big argument with two different doctors about a throat culture. This one included one doctor asking, "What makes you competent to judge a medical question?" and ended with the other doctor asking, "Do you refuse this treatment?" When I answered in the affirmative, they both fairly ran into the doctors' private conference room, closing the door more loudly than necessary.

I was becoming very uncomfortable about being the bad parent on the ward. It was obvious that every disagreement went down on the record, and that each new doctor read the record upon arrival. John went around behind me having friendly talks with the residents about their life stories, and I also tried to be appreciative of their patience and flexibility. But I began to wonder if, really, I was mostly a pain in the neck, disrupting the doctors over trivia.

But each time Rodney came on the ward he reassured me that I was doing exactly the right thing by being Sierra's constant advocate. Rodney confirmed that each test I had refused had been unnecessary. He assured me that these young residents were learning a great deal from us about how to work with parents, so I shouldn't feel too apologetic. The morning after my biggest confrontation with the two irate doctors, Rodney came striding in, grinning, direct from reading the record, and said, "Between you and me, you were right. No throat culture was necessary. There was nothing new to be discovered." I felt a huge surge of gratitude and relief. I had come to love Rodney's daily visits. They kept me on track, continuing to think, supported in the parental role that seemed so essential to me.

I felt I was modeling something important for Sierra: no abdication, constant thinking, maintaining some judgment over what happened to her, but still cooperating fully with the important tests and treatments and helping her face the "hard parts."

At the end of her stay, she had integrated the experience so well that her comment in answer to my question, "How do you feel about the hospital?" was, "I love the hospital. It has pretty flowers on the wall and lots of friendly people. The only thing I don't like is the hard parts." Two days after we had gotten home, she said, "In the hospital I do all the ne . . . neces . . . necessary hard things. But I don't do the things that aren't necess . . . necessary."

We discovered in this hospitalization that the support of Sierra's young friends was important to her. When her first round of agony ended, she got on the phone and called Annie (four years), Naveed (four years), Jonathan (four years), Rafe (seven years), and Nicole (nine years), to tell them all about her experiences. She did not want to talk to any grown-ups. When we left the hospital, we went directly to see her classmates at school.

When it all was over Sierra had no apparent emotional scars, except perhaps, a temporary desire to return to the hospital because, we guessed, she had received one hundred percent, twenty-four hour a day, two-parent attention for five days.

During this crisis I developed huge love for Rodney. It was so painful to be the nuisance parents. His reassurance meant the world to us.

It was consequently very upsetting when we learned that Rodney could not be the attending physician for Sierra's heart surgery at New York University Hospital because he did not have any affiliation there. We would have to work with someone who hardly knew us. This was particularly scary because Rodney had told us that when Sierra was eighteen months old, he was sure she would be a disaster due to our unusual form of parenting. After all, he told us, nobody else would ever let an eighteen-month-old decide if she were ready for an immunization, as we had. But by the time Sierra was three, he thought our parenting had been very successful because Sierra was already such a fine child. As a result, he had stopped forcing immunizations on toddlers as he used to.

But what would a new doctor, dealing with us for the first time, think of us? I dreaded the thought of going through heart surgery without Rodney. The idea of working with a doctor who disapproved of our parenting gave me the shudders.

Hopefully, Rodney would be able to provide the opening wedge into the other doctor's respect. Maybe he would tell Dr. Doyle that we were really okay. Maybe he would tell her that our ideas might seem weird, but they worked well in practice.

CHAPTER FOUR

Sierra Learns of the Coming Operation

On December 6, 1979, when Sierra was three and a half, I told her about the surgery. I had been wondering when I would tell her. I wanted her to be aware that someday she would have an operation, just as a matter of fact. No big deal, no big secret, no big anxiety—just a little piece of reality that we would share with her.

One cold Wednesday, after school, I was driving Sierra and her friend Naveed home in the car. I had just asked Sierra to sit in the back to keep Naveed company, since his parents didn't allow him to sit in front in case of an accident.

Naveed said, "If a car crashes then the car has to go to the shop."

"And the people probably have to go to the hospital," I remarked. I was not thinking about Sierra yet, but I wanted to extend Naveed's concern to include people as well as his beloved cars.

"Yeah," Sierra said. "People go to the hospital when it hurts very much or when it's cut and bleeding."

"Yes," I added. "That's true. People only go to the hospital when it hurts very very very much and when they don't know what's wrong and they need to find out." I was thinking of Sierra's stay at Lenox Hill. "Or sometimes," I continued, thinking of a car accident, "when it hurts and they do know what's wrong and they need to fix it." Then it dawned on me that Sierra's situation was different. I added, "And sometimes when it doesn't hurt but there's something wrong that needs to be fixed—like Annie's hernia. It didn't hurt her, but she had a lump that needed to be taken out."

"Yeah," Sierra said, "and now Annie has a little scar there."

"Yes," I said, "like, Sierra, you'll probably go to the hospital some day and have an operation to fix your heart so that it doesn't go *boom-boom-sshhhh. boom-boom-sshhhh.*"

Sierra seemed only slightly taken aback. She turned after a two second interval to Naveed and said, "Did you know my heart goes *boom-boom-sshhh*? *Boom-boom-sshhh*?" She had a little smile on her face and an intense look of someone sharing an important thing.

I looked at Naveed. "Yes," I said, "most people's hearts go *boom-boom, boom-boom*, but Sierra's heart goes *boom-boom-sshhhh, boom-boom-sshhhh* because she has a little narrow place in her blood vessel. They'll have to fix it to let the blood flow smoothly."

"When we went to the hospital they thought I had a her . . . a *what*?" Sierra asked me.

"An appendicitis. That's when there's an infection in your appendix and they have to take it out."

"Yeah," Sierra went on, "when you have many, er, white blood cells they know you have an infection."

"That's right," I said. "When you have more white blood cells in your blood than usual they know you have an infection."

"There are also red blood cells. My Daddy says there are many kinds of cells. All different kinds," Sierra was sharing her new knowledge from Lenox Hill.

"Yes, your whole body is made of all different kinds of cells. You know what a cell is like? It's very very tiny and it's something like an egg."

Naveed chimed in now that we were back on familiar ground. "Sometimes ducks hatch from eggs. And we eat them. Sometimes chickens do. And we eat chickens too."

Sierra carried the conversation on to its logical conclusion: "And we also eat turkeys."

I parked the car, and we moved on to something else. I was excited by the conversation. It seemed like the most natural way in the world to give Sierra this information. It had again worked well to talk with her and a friend. She had taken the new information in stride, related it to the familiar thing about her heart's odd sound, and the familiar experience at Lenox Hill. The information had registered. I felt I would soon overhear her telling someone that she was going to have an operation to fix her heart.

CHAPTER FIVE

We Inform and Confuse Ourselves

By Christmas vacation, 1979, the pace of our concern over the operation had quickened. Even though we had both been extremely busy, the Lenox Hill experience had forced our attention to the issue.

We went to visit Judy Lamar, a high school classmate I had met again at my twentieth high school reunion. She had told me at the reunion that she was a pediatrician, and that she had studied to be a pediatric cardiac surgeon. I was delighted. Somehow knowing someone in that field seemed like a magical opening to learn everything. She told me she had books she would lend me. Rodney had told us in the fall that it was time we started preparing for the operation. He had said he would lend us his library privileges so we could go and read the literature and become informed.

He had also told us that it would take about a year of negotiations with the hospital administration to get permission to be in the recovery room, which of course he thought we should do. He had advised us to send a letter to Dr. Doyle telling her all our concerns, and including all the writing I had previously done about Sierra and doctors.

We had not done any of this. As a result, I was beginning to feel uneasy about being behind. After all, Dr. Doyle wanted to see us again in January. It was now December, and we had made no progress except for our experience at Lenox Hill. Really, if we wanted Dr. Doyle to get to know us, we should have written her before our January visit!

Worse still, I had just been informed that the $500,000 proposal I had written for the Youth Action Program to run a leadership school and a network of Homes Away From Home for homeless teenagers, had been funded by the Federal Government, requiring the pace of my work to triple, draining me completely, just when I should be turning my attention to Sierra. Deep down I didn't want the grant. I wanted to take care of my family, and I knew the grant represented overextension even in the best of times. But I had to take it on. I felt I had a moral commitment to all the teenagers in our project to go full steam ahead, creating as much forward movement as possible. I had a dream of a youth movement, taking responsibility for the community, and I was committed to doing the necessary work. But the prospect of the coming year made me extremely anxious.

It was wonderful to see my high school classmate. She encouraged us to educate ourselves. "You are educated people," she said, "There's no way that you can give up your need to know. Read everything, master the literature. Don't abdicate to the medical profession."

I thought she was somewhat overstating our need to know, based on her own intense intellectual curiosity.

Nonetheless, her encouragement was good. She gave us a huge pile of pediatric cardiology books. The pile was three feet high, weighing about thirty pounds. I was thrilled.

John hid the books from Sierra, putting them in the trunk of the car. She was asleep in the car. We hadn't told her the purpose of our visit.

When we got to my parents' house, I carried in the books. John said with some urgency, "Please low-profile the books."

I started to carry them into the living room, saying to my mother, "Look what Judy gave us .... !" But John stopped me, grabbing my arm. "Stop. Please don't make a big deal out of these books." He was vehement. So I stopped. We had a hot little discussion. Suddenly he seemed very worried, not trusting me, afraid I was going to communicate worry to Sierra.

It seemed to me that he was up against the slight denial I felt he had, that is, he hadn't wept much, hadn't worried much, hadn't even thought about it much. He said, "I don't want Sierra to see us poring worriedly over a huge stack of books as if it were a big, big, deal." I said, "I'm not going to pore worriedly, just read avidly, and I don't plan to tell her what exactly the books are for, but if it seems appropriate I don't think it would hurt to say something like, 'Yes, these books tell all about the body and the heart and I'm going to read them so I can understand what the doctors tell me and I can understand exactly what is going to happen when we take you for your heart operation.' "

I did agree with John that there was no reason to do that now, nor to have a whole year of active anticipation—two months would probably be plenty. But I thought secrecy, or any air of forbidden subjects, would be the worst; the next worst would be John and me arguing about it. I quieted my eagerness to show the books and set them unobtrusively on a table in the back room. I realized that this kind of disagreement was just part of the whole picture. It undoubtedly would not be the last time John and I exchanged some hot words about how to handle it.

Right after our Christmas visit to my parents in the Boston suburbs, John's mother called with fear in her voice and heart. She said, "John, your father is dying, and I need your help. I don't think he'll live another week. I think it would be best if you flew out here right away, before it's too late."

John's parents live outside of Seattle. He agreed to go. I insisted, "If you're going to leave for a week right now, just when we've received this grant and my work pace is stepping up, you've got to take Sierra with you. I can't take time off from work."

He agreed that Sierra could go along. That meant she would be having deep family experience, focused on sickness, dying, and maybe even death. She seemed perfectly able to handle it. The night before they left, as John and I were struggling to explain the situation, saying "John's father is very sick . . . " Sierra interrupted, saying, "You mean he's dying? He might die? John's going out there to help his mother and I'm going along. That's okay." She was three and a half years old!

They flew to Seattle, leaving me with my cardiology books. I began reading them at night, late, after midnight, sitting up in bed or at my desk, poring over these books.

I went right for the scary parts. I read about all the possible complications of the coarctation operation. I read, for example, about acute bacterial endocarditis, which is an infection of the wound; and about an aneurism at the site of the stitches in the aorta if too much tension is on the aorta; and about danger to the gastrointestinal tract. I read about how the dye in the angiogram used during the catheterization to locate the precise spot of the coarctation can kill patients if it is wrongly used.

This was all somewhat disturbing. But the worst of all came on page 801 of *Congenital Malformations of the Heart*. It said:

> Coarctation occurs far more frequently in males than in females. The reason for this sex difference is not known. It is, however, a striking fact that boys with coarctation of the aorta show precocious physical development. In contrast, the condition is rare among women of normal physical development, but as reported by Albright et al. and Wilkings and Fleishmann, it occurs frequently among women with ovarian agenesis. Wilkins has found that these 'women' carry the male sex chromosome. Thus, it is possible that the etiological factor in this malformation is related to or carried in the male sex chromosome.

I didn't know what it meant. I didn't know what ovarian agenesis was. I guessed it meant women who had no eggs and therefore couldn't have babies. After all, the meaning of ovarian was clear; and agenesis had to mean something like no birth, no beginning. Then putting the word "women" in quotation marks! What did that mean?

I thought of all the wonderful conversations Sierra and I have about how she will grow up and have a baby that will come out of her uterus like she came out of mine and she will be a mother, like I am. I realized how deeply I had been implanting that idea. I thought I had better start saying things more like, "Some women have babies, but some women don't have babies . . . you might decide you want to, or you might not . . ." Something more neutral so she would not get disappointed if she has this "ovarian agenesis."

The next morning, fortunately, I had scheduled a co-counseling session with my friend Tom Roderick. This meant we would listen to each other talk about our feelings, taking turns for forty-five minutes each. In my turn I cried and cried about Sierra not being able to have babies. And, of course, I thought I had better start having more babies myself if she were to be sterile. It grew even more disturbing. As I started thinking about Sierra having a male sex chromosome, I started imagining her with a beard, without proper breasts, and I got upset. I visualized her as a bearded teenager looking wistfully at the lovely feminine picture of herself at three and a half.

I carried around this deeply uneasy feeling about Sierra until John and Sierra got home on January 12th. But three days passed before I had a private minute with John just before we went to sleep.

"John, there's something I need to tell you."

Hearing my tones, he asked, "Is it something I would want to sleep on?"

I replied, "I've been sleeping on it for a week."

"Well," he said, "don't tell me now unless you need to. Save it for tomorrow."

I figured I could hold off one more day, so he went to sleep. I stayed awake, tossing and turning, thinking about all the issues that needed attention at work. Only when it occurred to me to get up and write some notes about Sierra did I realize what was really keeping me awake.

The operation was always somewhere in my mind. Anything in the future would have to wait for the operation to be over. I couldn't have another baby until Sierra was safe. I couldn't take on any new responsibilities until this was over. I felt a panic about my work because I couldn't handle both.

Whenever I looked at Sierra, I would imagine the big scar. I would imagine them breaking her ribs. If she were dancing, I would wonder if she would have a long recovery before she would dance again. If she were smiling at me,

I'd be wondering if she would have brain damage after the operation.

Reading the cardiology books had impressed me with how small the working space is around a person's aorta—especially a child's aorta. Somehow, I had imagined the coarctation to be a little further away from the heart, not all tangled up in the aortic arch and all the major arteries leading off it. There seemed much more room for error than I had thought.

I stayed up several hours that night making notes, reading more cardiology texts and worrying.

The next morning, I still didn't have a chance to talk to John alone. Since Sierra was living in our room with us, we really had very little privacy. Once the day began, usually with Sierra saying, "Mommmmy!" it was always a big rush until evening. Then, since Sierra also usually stayed up until about eleven, John and I didn't get much time in the evening. It was a good thing we believed in including Sierra in family life, because if we had been eager to get her to sleep at seven or eight, we would have been insanely frustrated. From the moment she was born she needed only eleven hours of sleep a day. When she was five it was down to about nine.

That evening, John, Sierra, and I went downstairs to Tom and Maxine's apartment to talk to Tom. He had been to the hospital that day for a barium enema. We were taking every opportunity to let Sierra talk with people about hospital experiences.

Sierra asked, "Did you have soapy water in your enema?"

Tom replied, "No, mine was just white fluid." He was laughing with embarrassment. It was not Tom's style to talk about his enemas with the public.

I asked, to keep the conversation going, and knowing that Sierra would be interested in this question, "Did they just do it once?"

"No, twice," he said.

"I had it three times!" Sierra bragged.

I corrected her. "Really only twice."

Tom, good teacher that he is, said, "It felt like three times right, Sierra?"

Sierra moved on to the real question. "Did you have a board on your arm for the IV?"

"No, I had no IV."

"I had to stay in the hospital for four days," Sierra went on.

"I just stayed for two and a half hours," Tom replied. The conversation continued a few more minutes. These conversations about medical things were always very interesting to us. We listened to find out what was really on her mind, what she had understood, what was worrying her, if anything. Usually, there was no great revelation, but it seemed like progress to us that medical conversations were part of her life, that her experience at Lenox Hill had given her enough knowledge to talk to grown-ups about their experiences. She wouldn't be too scared of the unknown when it came to hospitalization again.

Later that evening Tom and Maxine came upstairs to talk some more with us. Sierra had gone to bed early. Tom was concerned about whether he was getting cancer, or colitis, but in either case the persistent pain in his colon had alarmed him about his tension-producing lifestyle.

When Tom and Maxine left, we remained. I snatched the first opportunity I'd had in several days to tell John about page 801 and ovarian agenesis:

> John, here's what I wanted to tell you last night. I've been reading the cardiology books. I found a passage that said coarctation is extremely rare among girls and when it occurs in girls, it's often associated with something called 'ovarian agenesis'. Now, I don't know what that means, but it sure sounds like she can't have any babies. But then the book also said that it was associated with the male sex chromosome, and referred to the women who had it in quotes. As if they weren't really women. That's what I wanted to tell you.

John's reaction was strong. He was alarmed, it seemed, more than any time before about the surgery. "My God," he said, "A freak! Does that mean she'll grow a beard? Does a male chromosome mean male hormones? Oh, no." His sense of humor returned, and with a small smile, he said, "A monster. We've created a monster. A bearded ballet dancer with breasts. Well, if that's true there's nothing we can do about it. Maybe it means she doesn't have ovaries. Well, let's find out. Let's get to see Dr. Doyle." He put his arms around me, and we both cried for a few minutes.

"Maybe we can't have another baby," I said. "Maybe there's something wrong with our genes." I realized I assumed the problem was John's genes, of course, and I wondered if the reverse was in his mind, but I decided not to ask. Then I thought maybe it was my age, since I was thirty-four when Sierra was born. I started worrying about whether we should ever have another baby since I'll be even older! Then it passed through my mind that probably the baby I hadn't had, the abortion I'd had, would have been perfectly healthy. My mind zoomed on. I became aware that if I hadn't spent many hours sobbing out this old guilt and loss in co-counseling sessions, I would have interpreted Sierra's problem as punishment for my having had an abortion. Fortunately, this entered my mind only as a faint thought, not an overwhelming sense of guilt. I have, over the years, cried and raged and gotten out so much guilt, loss and anger that I'm pretty free of it nowadays. That abortion was the one thing in my life I deeply regretted, and it used to plague me in the form of an irrational conviction that I was bound to die young of a degenerative disease because I abdicated responsibility for what would have been my firstborn. Thank God, I thought, for co-counseling. I'd hate to be blaming myself these days for Sierra's heart anomaly!

John and I finished our conversation, agreeing to get some accurate information as quickly as possible.

The next day I called Rodney to ask him. His secretary called back to say that Rodney knew of no such connection between coarctation and ovarian agenesis, but he would research it over the weekend, if I would tell him what book I found the information in.

In the evening, we had dinner with Sierra's friend Naveed and his family. Naveed's mother, Claude, told me Naveed had said he "wanted to grow up to be a mommy." Sierra said, "I'm going to be a mommy, right?" And I responded, in my first clumsy effort to give her a more neutral sex role identification, "Yes, . . . but . . . you might change your mind . . ."

During this period, I started waking up in the night with heart palpitations of my own. Fear was getting a hold of me. It seemed to be a combination of work responsibilities and fear for Sierra. I made an appointment with Dr. Steven Lam, our regular doctor, just to check my own heart.

He said, "I can't find anything wrong. Your blood pressure is fine. Your pulse is fine. Are you worrying about something?"

Of course I was. I asked him, "What do you know about ovarian agenesis? I read in the cardiology books that coarctation of the aorta is associated in girls with ovarian agenesis, but I don't know what it is."

"It is very unlikely that Sierra would have that. There are usually other symptoms. I would advise you to stop reading the cardiology books. An educated consumer is dangerous in the area of medicine. You had better find a doctor you trust, and trust him."

I left Dr. Lam's office somewhat relieved, but not convinced that I should stop trying to educate myself. I felt I had no choice but to be an educated consumer. I could not abdicate my ability to try and understand. I realized that no matter how much I tried there would be unexpected and incomprehensible things, but Judy's and Rodney's encouragement to learn felt more supportive than Dr. Lam's caution.

While there I asked Dr. Lam, since he is associated with New York University Medical Center, if he knew the surgeons who did pediatric cardiac surgery. He said, "Dr. Wayne Isom is the one who is doing most of the pediatric cardiac surgery. He is the best. I recommend him. Either him or Dr. Spencer. They are both excellent."

Suddenly the prospect of our having to choose surgeons was before me. I had assumed there was one best one, and we would get him. Now there were two, and we would have to choose. But then I remembered that Judy Lamar had told us that all the pediatric cardiac surgeons are at the very top of the medical fields because there is no room for error.

The rest of January and February and most of March passed quickly, with John and me mostly engrossed in work. We decided that even though we had not written Dr. Doyle a letter yet, we had better go see her, since she had suggested January.

On March 20th we went to see Dr. Doyle for the second time. On the way to her office, in the car, I said to Sierra, "You know, Sierra, Dr. Doyle is the person who will tell us when you need your heart operation. That's why we're going to see her."

"Why do I have to have an operation?"

"Because if you don't fix your heart it will be bad for your body as it grows. You'll get very bad headaches and other things.

Why don't you ask Dr. Doyle? She knows everything about it. She's the one who told us you would have to have an operation."

At the office, Sierra listened intently and asked a few factual questions about the model of the heart. When Dr. Doyle asked Sierra to sit on the examining table, Sierra got very earnest. She was concentrating all her attention on being good. Her face was so sweet, so intent, as she watched every move Dr. Doyle made and held herself very still for blood pressure and pulse tests in both arms and legs.

John and I stood back, arms entwined, watching with infinite pride and concern. Sierra is such a beautiful child, in every way.

After the examination, Dr. Doyle again ran it down to us:

> Sierra has a moderately severe coarctation of the aorta which requires surgery between the age of four and five. They used to wait until age eight or ten to do these

> operations, but the delay could cause irreversible damage to her blood vessels due to the high blood pressure. It's an operation that has been done well for twenty years. We've never lost a patient at this hospital. The mortality rate is two percent, but that applies primarily to infants where there are other difficulties. Ordinarily a catheterization is done first, to identify the exact location of the coarctation. This can be done during the same hospitalization as the surgery itself, or it can be done in advance. That's up to you. The catheterization involves hospitalization for two days. The surgery will be about ten days all together. I suggest we do the catheterization this May and the operation during the summer.

Yikes! She was speeding it up. That was too soon for us. But it brought home the point that the time was coming. "No," one of us said, "we can't do it that quickly. We would prefer to do it in the fall." Having the summer between us and it was more comfortable.

"All right," she said. "We'll be in touch when the time comes closer. I'll need six weeks' notice to schedule it."

"Dr. Doyle, we have one more question. We read that coarctation is sometimes associated with ovarian agenesis. Is that anything to be concerned about?"

"Not at all," she said. "Not in Sierra's case. She has no secondary symptoms whatsoever."

We left, again relieved. As we crossed First Avenue, Sierra asked, "When do I have to have an operation? Is it going to be soon?"

"No," we said. "Not for quite a while."

"Good," Sierra said," "I don't want it soon."

CHAPTER SIX

Sierra Gets Ahead of Us

WE AGAIN PUT IT out of our minds for a while. But on May 2nd Sierra and I happened to offer Annie and Judy Thoms a ride home after school. It turned out that they were going to visit a friend of Annie's named Sasha who had just had open heart surgery and was home from the hospital. As we drove up Broadway, I said to Annie, "Sasha had an operation something like the one Sierra is going to have, except it's different in one way. Sasha's operation was actually inside her heart, and Sierra's is going to be outside her heart, just in the aorta."

Annie was surprised. "Sierra's going to have an operation?" Judy hadn't told Annie that Sierra would have an operation because she wasn't sure if Sierra knew yet.

I asked if we could go with Annie and Judy, so Sierra could meet Sasha.

As we crossed the street, Sierra took my hand tightly. We both knew this approaching meeting with Sasha had taken on importance.

Sasha's door was opened by a very pregnant woman. Annie yelled, "Sasha!" A child Annie's age zoomed out from the back room, down the long corridor, right up to us, with a huge, welcoming smile. She said, "Come on, Annie." And she zoomed back down the corridor.

Sierra went to the back room for a couple of minutes with Sasha and Annie. I turned to Sasha's mother, "Sierra is going to have heart surgery next fall. We would love to get together some time and talk about it. We would like to hear everything you went through, from start to finish, and what we should look out for."

"We'd love to do that," Julie said. "It was a hard year for us—this operation was hanging over Sasha's head for a whole year. Sometime let's get some babysitters so we can talk privately, and we'll tell you all about it."

Sierra and I didn't stay more than five minutes. But that was long enough for Sierra, and me, to be reassured.

On the way down in the elevator Sierra said, "She sure is zooming around the house! Like this!" She held out her pointing finger and made a zipping motion all around the air in front of her. She giggled. She was obviously impressed and seemed relieved as well.

At dinner I said to John, "We visited Sasha today. Sasha is Annie's friend." I waited to see if Sierra would add anything. John knew from my tone that there was something important here, so he asked, "You visited Sasha, Sierra?" Sierra was silent. She was clearly reluctant to speak, so we moved on to other topics. Her reluctance was unusual. She seemed already to have invested this relationship with considerable energy.

About ten minutes later she reopened the conversation spontaneously, "Sasha had a heart operation but she was zooming around her apartment, like this!" She made her little zipping hand motion again, with a little smile. That's all she chose to say.

A week later we visited Rodney because Sierra had an ear infection. I remarked, "Last week we met a girl Sierra's age who had a heart operation."

"That's wonderful! Just let them alone together. Don't worry what they're doing. Peer support is very important."

Sierra said, "Yeah, she had a heart operation, and she was zooming around!" She again made the little hand motion, "like that!"

"Otherwise," I said, "all our great resolutions about preparation are kind of in abeyance. I've been too busy to do anything."

"No," Rodney said. "You're doing well. You've found peer support. That's important."

Sierra had started humming and singing, seemingly deliberately to drown out our conversation. I said, "Sierra knows about the operation and is getting ready for it." I looked at her, "Right?"

She smiled a secret knowing little smile, and said very quietly, "Right."

We stopped the conversation.

Three days later, on Sunday morning, Sierra woke up and said, "Today I want to go to Sasha's house. More than any other thing, I want to play with Sasha." I was surprised. Again, it was clear that the contact mattered.

The next day Sierra and Sasha spent the afternoon together. We did as Rodney suggested. Just left them alone. Heaven knows what communication occurred, but we know there was a lot. They played operation all afternoon. They examined Sasha's great big curvy scars under what would be her breasts. Sierra and Sasha spent an afternoon together every other weekend all spring. Soon, hospital play took over all Sierra's relationships. We stayed out of it. We saw no indication of worry emerging from it.

After our very careful buildup, introducing the idea of an operation so gradually, we let go of control over the communication and turned it over to a five-year-old who had already had a similar experience, who was zooming around her house with confidence and zest.

By June 29th, Sierra was ready to discuss her operation on the most direct and serious level with adults.

We had joined several other families in renting a summer house on the New Jersey shore. Some of these families were old friends; most were new acquaintances. The second Friday night, when we all gathered around the dinner table, we each took turns telling about our week. It was a way to get to know each other, and to touch base after a hard week's work.

Of course, we gave the children each a turn, although not all of them chose to speak. It can be very intimidating to have ten adults waiting to hear what you're going to say. When it was Sierra's turn, with all eyes upon her, she announced, "I am going to have a heart operation." That was it. She had no more to say. She left the table.

One of our new acquaintances in that summer vacation home turned out to be a child psychiatrist. He and I spent the remainder of the dinner time talking about the operation. He told me that the catheterization would be the most frightening for Sierra. "She will be conscious during the catheterization. They don't give general anesthesia. She'll just be sedated. She'll know what's going on and be helpless to stop it. If you're not there, it'll be very scary. You should insist on being there no matter what."

I knew that John and I would probably faint if we had to witness doctors making an incision in Sierra's groin and inserting a tube up into her heart. I really did not want to be present. But this image the psychiatrist was painting of Sierra conscious and terrified, sedated but aware, convinced me.

Once convinced, however, I was not better off. I didn't feel confident that we could deal with the big-time doctors who do heart surgery. How could we insist on being present for the catheterization? To whom would we insist? Sierra's cardiologist is so impressive and so very professional. We're not even on a first-name basis with her. I don't have the time to figure it all out and work my way through this maze. I wouldn't need so much time if we just went along with Dr. Doyle's program. But if we're going to try and break any new ground, as both Rodney and now this other doctor are encouraging us to do, it would take something more.

Later that evening Sierra was sitting on my lap as we listened to John and Olin, our new psychiatrist friend, play guitar and banjo. Her attention was still on the operation. She whispered to me, "Will I have a scar?"

"Yes . . . How do you feel about that?"

"I like the scar . . . it's the knife I don't like."

"You probably won't even see the knife. You'll be unconscious." "Well," she explained. "It's not the knife . . . it's the cutting I don't like."

Well, that's to the point, I thought. I guess she knows what she doesn't like! Since I was speechless on that point, Sierra went on. "Does the thing they use to make me unconscious have a funny smell?"

"I don't know. Let's ask Olin. He's a doctor."

Soon we began getting reports from other people that Sierra was announcing to everyone that she would soon have a heart operation. She was getting various reactions, from what I could find out, and I hoped nobody was reacting with too much alarm. I knew that when she told Celeste, the mother of her two best teenage friends, Celeste said, "Oh, no! Not you! You don't need an operation. You're so healthy." Jenny told me she tried to improve on her mother's reaction by saying, "I'm sure it's necessary for you to have an operation or your parents wouldn't agree to have it."

In any case, by summer Sierra had clearly integrated a lot of information and accepted the idea that she would have an operation. It was good that she was opening up conversation about it.

By midsummer she was way ahead of us. As we drove with two of our close East Harlem teenagers, Freddy and Jenny, to Cape Cod for a weekend on August 2nd, Sierra swung around to sit on the little seat between the driver and the front seat passenger. She turned toward Jenny and Freddy and launched into earnest conversation about Mary Poppins. Then, seemingly out of the blue, she made her pronouncement, "I'm going to have a heart operation. I'll have a big scar like Sasha's only not exactly like hers. Mine is going to be on one side. It's going to be pretty soon—when I go back to Calhoun—in September. But I have a couple of days."

John and I nearly gasped. Sierra was planning to have the operation in a couple of days! In September! She's way ahead of us, we thought. We haven't gotten anything planned yet. We haven't taken time to prepare ourselves and schedule anything or get to know the exact procedure or even sit down with Sasha's parents.

We've only taken the time to prepare Sierra, and now she's ready and we're not!

This triggered a lot of discussion between John and me during the weekend. We were staying in a tiny cottage that belonged to a friend of my mother's, along Manomet Bluff in Massachusetts. The cottage looked out over a huge cliff, down onto the beach. It was a glorious view, and a cozy cottage. We crammed our extended family into it, with Freddy and Jenny, and our friend Tim Parsons who came from Boston to be with us.

Each morning Freddy, Jenny, and Tim went down over the bluff to swim and explore. They took Sierra with them, leaving John and me free to consult and to counsel.

Up to now I haven't explained much about this "co-counseling" that we do. I think I should, since it plays such a critical part in our preparations. Co-counseling is a way for people to get together in pairs and give each other undivided attention, assisting each other in unloading the feelings of hurt, anger, grief, fear, embarrassment, boredom, frustration, despair, and whatever other pain a person may have. The theory is that all of us were born wonderful—loving, intelligent, cooperative, eager for life. The extent to which we don't act that way all our lives is precisely the extent to which we've been hurt, physically or emotionally, along the way. But, according to the co-counseling theory, it is possible to recover from those hurts and regain our full potential for living. The key to doing so is having a safe enough context, supported by nonjudgmental people who help us get relief from the weight of painful emotion. Relief comes in the form of emotional catharsis: laughing, crying, raging, trembling, and nonrepetitive talking. This form of catharsis gives enough relief so we can begin to change the behavior patterns that are getting in the way of our lives, and we can think more clearly about the difficult situations we face in the present, without being overly influenced by confusing feelings from the past.

The way it's done is this: two people get together and exchange thirty to forty-five minutes each of undivided attention. The counselor listens, completely supporting whatever the counselee needs to say or feel. The counselor makes no judgment, gives no opinion or advice, but simply encourages the counselee to stick with the points that are most emotion-laden, and let the feelings flow out. There is trust that each of us has the ability to heal ourselves and move on to healthier outlooks, as long as we get that necessary support from another human being who cares. Of course, for experienced co-counselors the process becomes more complex and we develop more skill, as we try to battle our way out of deeply ingrained patterns of irrational behavior and feeling. Relief is not the only goal—changing ourselves is the more profound one, to act always in the most thoughtful, rational, and caring way possible. But lots of very good co-counseling occurs with relief as the main immediate outcome. Once relieved, people are naturally able to act more in keeping with their best ideas and values, and less reactively.

John and I co-counsel like this regularly, with each other and with our friends. It isn't just a casual thing we invented ourselves. Both of us were certified teachers of Re-evaluation Counseling, which is the more formal name for co-counseling. We have long belonged to an international network of people who help each other in this way.

We joined a class in co-counseling in 1972 when our relationship seemed to be on the rocks. That was two years before we married. Janet Pfunder, a college classmate of mine, kept telephoning to say, "I'm doing this great thing called Re-evaluation Counseling. I'm starting a class and I would love to have you join it." We said, "No," about five times until one night she called us when we were racking our brains about what to do with each other. We were stuck, where relationships always get stuck, up against the difficult parts of each other that would not seem to yield to reason or anger. John was periodically confessing to me that he couldn't love me or anyone enough to make a commitment. I was mortally wounded, depressed, and angry, each time. When I had finally, at age thirty, opened myself up to trust someone enough to marry him, I was being rejected. I didn't really believe him, because it seemed to me from the way he treated me that he did love me, and that his idea that he couldn't love anybody was just a symptom of his not having easy access to his deepest feelings. Nonetheless, I did a lot of unhelpful sulking and blaming.

When Janet called one evening in October, we said, "Why not. We obviously need some help to get out of this quagmire.

We don't want to give up the relationship. Maybe somehow this co-counseling will help."

It did. Soon we were listening to each other's deepest feelings and helping each other in new ways. John was opening up on new levels. Things didn't seem stuck anymore. When we ran up against the same obstacles, we would co-counsel, and each of us would remember what the other one's deeper struggle was. This made it possible to keep loving. Guilt, hurt, and resentment became irrelevant. Something we called "re-emergence," meaning the full recovery of our true nature and rational intelligence, no longer obscured by early hurts—became more interesting.

Co-counseling enabled us to know each other as deeply as we could imagine without having to go through the terrible emotional and sometimes physical violence that people go through when they are deeply engaged and refuse to give up, but are embroiled in each other's irrational needs and fears. I had been through those before with other people. Tumultuous relationships bring people very close, oftentimes; but the scars are as deep as the involvement. John and I were grateful for having found a more gentle route to the same depth. The co-counseling route left no scars.

Naturally we had both begun co-counseling about Sierra's operation as soon as we learned about it. We figured the more and the earlier we dumped our own fears, guilts, and confusions, the better we would be able to handle Sierra's feelings.

Many of our friends told us that when they had operations the hardest thing for them was that their parents "freaked out." The actual experience would not have been so bad if their parents had not been terrified, or angry, or paralyzed, or absent. Or if their parents hadn't lied to them, or over-protected them, or assumed they were incapable of understanding what was happening to them. This made a lot of sense to us. The burden of not "freaking out" was ours. We wanted Sierra to know that when things got really rough, her parents would be right there with her: caring, rational, supportive, sharing, strong, open to her feelings, able to handle whatever came up. We believed this was at least as important to her overall development as a person, and to her relationship with us, as any other single thing we had faced together as a family.

It wasn't that we thought Sierra couldn't cope with whatever happened. Children have always coped, even when—especially when—their parents "freak out." But we didn't want Sierra to have to do that. We wanted to have an experience of gracefully handling major heart surgery in a way that made all of us proud, close, and happy. We wanted Sierra to emerge emotionally stronger, not weaker or more frightened, than before.

That morning at Manomet Bluff, John and I co-counseled together about Sierra. We both admitted that the idea of Sierra dying was on our minds a lot. When we let her go down into the foggy, foggy morning with Tim and Jenny, and heard them calling to each other, we both wondered if she would be lost in the ocean. When Jenny had her out on the bicycle at 11:30 p.m. we were both wondering if she would be killed. Whenever John or I look at her beautiful, tan, athletic, and coordinated little body, we are usually imagining the scar, or imagining the surgeon cutting through her side. We both cried a lot that morning.

Then we started talking. John thought we should take a light tone in all our discussions with her. "We should let her know we are not at all worried. It should be like an adventure with her body. An amazing thing that they know how to do the catheterization. Let's have tone of delight and wonder, not of worry."

"No," I said. "I think that's false, a little forced. Okay, some of it is amazing and wonderful. But our basic tone should be more matter of fact. There are parts that will be scary, parts unknown, parts we can't prepare her for. We need to be straightforward about all of it. No one tone is right. There's a lot happening."

This difference represented an ongoing difference between John and me. He generally reaches for the tips of the mountains and the wonderful life. I have my feet more sunk in the mud. The combination usually comes out about right. So we agreed to point out the wonder of it, but also to accept the scary parts, and generally to be pretty matter-of-fact.

We reminded ourselves that one thing we had learned at Lenox Hill was that we must prepare her for the unexpected. There will be surprises. No matter how hard we try to prepare, there will be surprises.

Then we made a long list of things we needed to do in preparation. At the top of the list was writing our big LETTER to Dr. Doyle. Writing it would get us clear on what it was we were asking of the hospital and the doctors.

By early September, it was written.

CHAPTER SEVEN

The Letter

September 14, 1980

Dr. Eugenie F. Doyle, M.D.
566 First Avenue
New York, NY 10016

Dear Dr. Doyle:

When you examined our daughter, Sierra Stoneman-Bell, this winter, you suggested that we go ahead with surgery for her coarctation sometime this fall, and that we do the catheterization first and separately. You also let us know that you would be on vacation in October and that you would need six weeks warning to schedule Sierra in the hospital and in your own schedule.

We have been so extremely and unusually busy this past year at work that we find ourselves way behind in our own preparations for the surgery. Although Sierra is well enough prepared that yesterday we overheard her telling friends that she would be having her operation "in September, in a couple of days," we ourselves need to back up and position ourselves to handle the experience in the best possible way, for her and ourselves and the medical team we will be working with.

We are now aiming for early November for the catheterization and January for the surgery.

As you may recall, in November 1979 we had an unexpected five-day stint in Lenox Hill Hospital while Sierra was tested for acute appendicitis. Those five days were an excellent preview for us. We all learned that we could handle that hospital experience with no ill effects. We learned something about our parental style in that situation; and we learned how critically important was the day-to-day support of our attending physician, Dr. Rodney Hite.

When we learned that Rodney would not be able to serve as the attending physician during the heart surgery, we got nervous about whether any doctor who hadn't gone through the past four years with us would be as sympathetic to our parental approach as Rodney has come to be.

Since you are the doctor most likely to play the role of overall guide,interpreter, and advocate, Rodney suggested that we write to you, being as clear and thorough as we can be about how we expect to approach the whole experience with Sierra and what we think we need from you. He also suggested that we send you the enclosed articles about Sierra's first 15 months and her early experiences with doctors. He was a little concerned, I think, because two years ago he thought our ways were a little odd. As he put it, "I thought

Sierra would turn out a disaster." But he has come to think that our decisions must have had some wisdom, since Sierra is doing so well. He feels, as we do, eager for us to establish the same level of trust and respect with the key person in the heart surgery that we have developed with him.

This letter is our first attempt to communicate what we are thinking so far about Sierra's experience as a cardiac patient. It's our first attempt to ask you if you can support our approach and if you have additional suggestions as to how we can implement it in practice.

First, what we think Sierra will need:

-She'll need one of us physically present, and oftentimes physically close, all of the time. Her own comments on her experience at Lenox Hill were that she wasn't scared as long as one of us was there; her only stated distress was not understanding why one of us suddenly left during the insertion of an intravenous needle (one of almost fainted when they had trouble finding the vein).

Some of the ramifications of this are obvious and acceptable in hospital practice: one of us will always sleep at the hospital, and we'll be there at every time allowable. Others we know are not so simple: Will she be conscious and can we be there during her catheterization? Can we be in the recovery room?

-She'll need full and detailed preparation about what to expect, step-by-step. She will need to have played it out, talked it out, seen as much of it as possible in advance, and met as many of the people involved as possible. We want to minimize surprises and prepare Sierra with the idea that there will be a few surprises, which we can identify when they come as the expected surprises.

The implications of this are not altogether clear to us: How can we get detailed enough knowledge? How can we be prepared for the hospital routines, all the different steps and test? Who is going to walk us through that process and when? Can we trust that the hospital will do this, or will you, or must we do independent research?

-She'll need ongoing respect for her ability to understand. She'll need things explained to her, as they happen, by us at the very least, but preferably by hospital personnel as well.

-She'll need to be able to cry and yell when things hurt or frighten her. We believe that emotional release is a critical part of human beings' ability to withstand, sort out, and recover from painful experience. We've seen Sierra many times go through something screaming at full lungs, but at the same time cooperating fully with the procedure.

The ramifications of this are fairly simple, for us and Sierra; but if the hospital personnel are constantly admonishing her not to cry, to be brave, strong, courageous and silent, we'll be at odds with them. We also need to make arrangements where we won't disturb the other patients.

-She'll need to retain some vestiges of power over her experience. There will need to be some areas of choice and decision, for her not to be forced to abdicate her usual sense of being in charge. Of course, there is the basic decision of whether or not to cooperate, and we are sure she will make that one. But beyond that, we found some little decisions in Lenox Hill were important: the decision not to wear a wristband because she wasn't going to the operating room; the decision not to have a rectal temperature taken because she hates it and it wasn't necessary; the decision not to have a blood test at a time when she was exhausted. These decisions were, by the way, important to us as well, enabling us to protect her in small ways from trivial trauma while she was mustering her full energy to handle the whole situation.

We think that one of the reasons she handled Lenox Hill so well was that she knew we had never abdicated our role as interpreters and protectors, occasionally warding off unnecessary procedures and insensitive personnel. As a result, her summary of her experience was, "I love the hospital. There are lots of friendly people and pretty wallpaper. The only thing I didn't like was the hard things I had to do … In the hospital I did the ne. . . ce . . . necessary things, but I didn't do the unnecessary things."

-She'll need maximum peer support. At least this means lots of telephone calls with her friends, lots of cards and little presents. We have located and she has developed a friendship with a five-year-old who had cardiac surgery last year, so she has already played out this friend's experience repeatedly and is familiar with the scar.

You allowed us to bring her best friend with her for her first examination. We need to explore whether there are any ways her friends can participate in her experience from here on. Can they visit? Can they make a preliminary tour with her to see the hospital? Can they come with her for explanations or play-outs of experience? Does the hospital provide this kind of preparation routinely or will we have to forge a preparatory path of our own?

As part of peer support, she'll need to make friends with other children on the ward. This will come easy for her, and we'll encourage it. But if there are other children her age scheduled to be on the ward during the same period, it would be good if it were possible to meet those children and families in advance, and perhaps visit each other's homes.

-She'll need competent and sensitive medical personnel at each stage.

-We think she'll need medical staff in the operating room who are willing to respect the hypothesis that patients actually hear and take in on some level of consciousness everything that is said around them while they are unconscious. While we can't prove this, we know there are indications in this direction. We think there is nothing to lose by assuming it to be true, and quite a bit to lose by ignoring it if it is true. Therefore, we want the opportunity to ask the surgical team to say only positive things about her, about her expected recovery, about the ease of repairing her aorta, and about what a strong and healthy child she is.

-She'll need us to feel confident and reasonably relaxed about what is going on.

Those are the general outlines of what we think Sierra will need. Of course, some of it reflects our own needs as well. In addition, there is something we expect to need as parents:

-We will need to set up our own network of peer support. This is obviously to help us, and is essentially in place.

We think the above pretty much covers the broad points on our minds. Do you think that if Sierra is scheduled for catheterization in early November that we have time between now and then to sort out and set up the situation consistent with the above points? Especially with your vacation coming up? Or should we wait and do it all in January and February?

We look forward to hearing from you.

Sincerely yours,

Dorothy Stoneman and John Bell
cc: Dr. Rodney Hite
Encl.

Enclosure to the letter:

SIERRA AND THE DOCTORS
Dorothy Stoneman

My first taste of agonized parental powerlessness came in the hospital, on the first day of Sierra's life outside my womb. The doctor came. She "examined" Sierra, by probing forcefully into her lower abdomen. When Sierra began to scream in pain and fear, the doctor shoved her thumb into Sierra's mouth to trigger her sucking reflex and thereby quiet her. She short-circuited Sierra's appropriate yelling response by forcing an inappropriate sucking response.

Perhaps there was no causal relationship, but seven weeks later Sierra began to show unspeakable terror when placed on her back to be changed. Seemingly from nowhere came absolute fear. She threw her arms out rigid, terror came into her face, and she shrieked. This went on for two days every time we lay her down. Finally, we were able to help her fully relieve this fear, with both of us lying next to her after she had been changed, talking reassuringly to her. She screamed and cried for 45 minutes. After that, her fear has never reappeared.

This period of being fearful happened to coincide with her first scheduled visit to the doctor for a shot. John decided to postpone the shot until the fear had passed.

When she did go for the shot, she was at a point (about nine weeks old) when she was often looking deeply into our eyes, trembling and reaching out with trust and excitement. Her whole tiny body was involved in this eye contact of love. Because it seemed reassuring, when John took Sierra to the doctor, he engaged her in this deep loving communication. While she looked trustingly into his eyes, the doctor pierced her leg with his needle. Sierra was stunned. That evening she cried and screamed for four solid hours, beginning again with the shriek of shock each time she met my eyes. It seemed for some days or weeks—that although she had relieved her immediate hurt, she didn't regain the absolute trust we had witnessed before.

The next time we went for a shot, I explained and warned her thoroughly and then sat a few feet away from her in the doctor's office and said, "Sierra, watch out! That person is going to give you a shot now and it will hurt!" Perhaps this was an overcompensation, but it seemed to work. When the shot was done, she cried for about two minutes and then returned to good spirits. The doctor was surprised. I thought her full emotional catharsis surrounding the pain and fear from the previous shot, as well as our consciously avoiding any violation of trust, had made this one easy.

When Sierra was fourteen months old, I had to take her all bundled up and miserable with a sore throat and fever to the doctor, who said he had to take a throat culture. This meant forcing Sierra on to her back, reaching into her sore throat and scraping for some germs. Although in her fever she didn't react much at the time, I think this was the beginning of a major fear of Rodney, the doctor. After this there was another visit in which Sierra had been frightened, but Rodney had moved in as doctors will and acted decisively to give her another shot.

The turning point came at our next visit, when Sierra was nineteen months. When Rodney passed through the waiting room, the terror came over Sierra. Seeing her fear, I decided never again to allow him to do anything to her without her agreement.

First the nurse tried coaxing and mildly bullying Sierra into getting weighed, measured, and her temperature taken. I mediated, offering Sierra the choice. She did choose to be weighed and measured, after twenty-five minutes of respectful explanation and demonstration. Then the doctor breezed in, armed with stethoscope and disarming smile. Sierra screamed and grabbed me. I assured her that I would not let the doctor do anything to her against her will. He was upset. He asked, "Does she respond this way with other people? Is this typical?" He said no other children ever responded to him this way . . . If they were scared, they were afraid of the table, or the needle, or the white coat, but not of HIM.

After having showed her how he listened to my heart, and offering Sierra a chance to listen to his (which she didn't), he seemed to feel he'd gone the limit, and he began moving in again. I told him she wasn't ready, but he kept coming. Finally, I physically pushed him away, saying, "NO! She's scared of you. I'm not going to abdicate my protective role just because you're a doctor. It's not necessary to listen to her heart at this moment." He backed away, and we talked. I insisted that all shots and examinations could now wait until she was old enough to understand and agree, when she had fuller verbal comprehension and knew that we were not just hurting her for nothing. He was very skeptical, but willing to experiment with the idea that maybe a child could understand if we waited.

So Sierra and I left, back in charge. It felt wonderful to have finally broken with the program. That night when John asked Sierra about her visit to the doctor she said, with intense pleasure, "Mommy said NO! Mommy said NO to Rodney!"

From nineteen months to twenty-two months we talked and talked about Rodney the Doctor. We read "Curious George Goes to The Hospital" about one hundred times, and every time we had a chance for intimate conversation Sierra would say, "Talk about Rodney." Over and over again we told all the stories, and acted out what happened at the doctor's office.

Then I made an appointment just for a special visit at Rodney's office. Sierra was eager to finally see him again, after all this preparation, but when we reached the office entrance, she went rigid and began to run crying to the street. I decided this was the point to move through fear, and explain some co-counseling theory. After letting her cry for a while, I explained that sometimes people feel afraid of things because of something that has happened before, but that when they know they are not really going to be hurt they learn how to act brave and do the scary thing even though they feel afraid; that it's OK to feel afraid and if she holds on tight to me we can go in together because I won't let her be hurt. She did decide to be brave, and, clinging tight, we went in.

This short visit was a complete success. Sierra left saying, "Rodney is my friend." When we returned for a real examination a month later, her terror of him was gone. But when he whizzed in, brandishing his stethoscope, obviously in no mood to indulge any further delays, she froze up and I again had to stop him: "Let me be the one to insist, or she'll be afraid of you again. Wait until she's ready." I explained to Sierra that she wasn't going to get a shot, but he was going to listen to her heart, and it wouldn't hurt. Reassured that we were still in charge, Sierra let Rodney listen to her heart while she cried and cried. She made no effort to stop him or squirm, nor did she hold back her yelling and crying and shaking. Then she smiled and let him look in her ears. She was over the hump.

On the next visit, at two years old, she let him give her a shot. She cried for about thirty seconds, and then began talking about it. We had many times acted out getting and giving shots with her close friend Annie who goes to the same doctor. We always screamed, "OUCH!" at the moment of being stuck, and then said, "It's better now." She was prepared. She knew what to expect, she knew it happened to other people, too, even to her friend Annie and to Curious George. The plan had worked—she was old enough to make her own decision, with enough information and confidence that she would not be made powerless.

Her comfort with doctors had remained. At two-and-a-half years, she had to go to a new doctor, who was very impressed with Sierra's calm willingness to follow all instructions, once she had established that she didn't want her temperature taken. This doctor said that two and a-half was usually "the worst age" for children and doctors, but Sierra was completely in charge and cooperative, since the doctor was respecting her right to say yes or no.

****

We enclosed two other articles along the same lines, the collection of which certainly gave Dr. Doyle a sense of our perspective and concerns.

On September 27th the phone rang. It was Dr. Doyle. "Mrs. Stoneman, I got your lo-o-ong letter."

I laughed nervously. She explained:

> Mrs. Stoneman, it is appropriate to be very concerned about the traumatic impact on children of hospitalization and surgery. Of course, we are all concerned about that. The staff at University Hospital are very sympathetic. Children are given dolls to act out what's done. They're given needles and syringes and what not.

> But you should know that the most traumatic part for a child is the needles. There will be things Sierra will not like. That cannot be avoided. The main thing is the shots. But, of course, each one will be explained and attempts to minimize the frequency will be made. Usually it all can be managed without trauma. You will be able to stay with her in the hospital except in the recovery room.

"But Mrs. Stoneman," she continued, "There is a tone in your letter . . . in fact I have underlined some sentences where you say you don't want Sierra to abdicate her usual feeling of being in charge." She chuckled. "You can't mean that a four-and-a-half-year-old is in charge."

"Well," I began kind of lamely, "she makes a lot of decisions . . . "

"Mrs. Stoneman, if she's in charge now you'll be in trouble when she's fourteen! You must understand that she will be a cardiac patient in the hospital for major surgery and she will not be in charge of anything. We deal with children and we try to make it nontraumatic. The main problem, as I said before, will be the needles. She will have a blood test at admission, a blood test at Bellevue within three weeks of the surgery to make sure she has no problems with clotting. There will be needles to sedate her prior to anesthetization. In the postoperative period she will have an intravenous line in for two days, and she will have a finger stick for hemoglobin test. I have tentatively set the catheterization for mid-November," she finished.

I didn't say much of anything in that conversation, except to keep suggesting that we make an appointment. It seemed to me that we should have a point-for-point discussion of the letter. At the end of the conversation we scheduled an appointment for October 21st.

After hanging up, I realized that we hadn't established the purpose of the October 21st meeting. I called back and learned from Dr. Doyle's secretary that she expected us to bring Sierra. That was not what I had in mind. I thought she should sit down with us at least once separate from Sierra, so we could talk freely about our anxieties. Always talking to the doctor with Sierra present was inhibiting.

I called back, and left the message that we wanted to come without Sierra. Her secretary confirmed the appointment for us alone.

Our visit with Dr. Doyle was completely satisfying. We went over every step of the catheterization, everything that would happen from the moment Sierra entered the hospital.

We were told that she would be admitted in the afternoon. Once on the ward she would be examined by an admitting intern or medical student. She would also be examined by a cardiac fellow. She'd be given an electrocardiogram, then be taken down for a chest x-ray on the second floor. She'd be asked to urinate in a cup. A lady would come and give her a finger stick to test her blood. Then she could go to the playroom.

She would have supper in bed. The nurses would take her temperature and her pulse regularly. One of us would sleep in a reclining chair. There would be a television and a telephone in the room.

After midnight Sierra would be allowed nothing to eat or drink, because the medication she would get in the morning sometimes causes an upset stomach.

At 8:30 a.m. she would be put on a rolling bed and carried to the catheterization room. She'd be put on the table there. A local anesthetic would be administered in her groin, then an incision made, the needle of the catheter inserted, and the tiny tube pushed up through her artery into her heart. An iodine dye, which makes a white image on the x-ray film, would be inserted, and then pictures would be taken of the dye moving through the heart.

The dye would be excreted through the kidney within fifteen minutes. There would be no aftereffects in her blood system. Children are tested in advance for a reaction.

Sierra could be shown the film of her heart on the TV monitor the next morning. The whole procedure would take an hour and a half. One catheter would be put through an artery and one through a vein. Blood would be drawn for the coagulation test during the catheterization in order to minimize the needles. Dr. Danilowicz would be in charge of the study, and Dr. Freedman and Dr. Lee would be there all the time. Dr. Doyle would move in and out of the room. Sierra would have a chance to meet all three doctors in advance.

Sierra would sleep most of the afternoon, and perhaps be sick a little with vomiting. By evening she would be fine.

Dr. Doyle would see her when she comes in, see her in the catheterization room, and would review the data and inform us of the findings before Sierra leaves.

Simple and straightforward as it was, all this information was a big relief. We finally had written down in our little notebooks everything we needed to explain to Sierra exactly what would happen to her.

We had two major decisions. John questioned the necessity of doing the catheterization. We had read unsettling things in our cardiology books. One book said patients should be warned that catheterization can have serious side effects, including death. Certain hospitals in Boston had a policy of not doing the catheterization at all, because of its risks.

Dr. Doyle was adamant on this point. She said the risks were in practice negligible. In twenty years, they had lost only one child, and that was a moribund infant. It was very important to do the test in advance to ensure that the surgery would not turn up more complications than expected. The time to find out about complications is not when the chest is open in front of the surgeon.

We went along with this. Somehow it seemed to me that if I were the surgeon, I would be pretty annoyed if parents denied me the fullest possible information about what I would have to repair once inside someone's body. I did not want to annoy the surgeon! I was reminded of all the parents of school children who used to say they didn't want to annoy their child's teacher because it might be taken out on the child. I always thought that was silly; no teacher would ever take it out on a child. But I found myself similarly loathe to alienate the person who would be handling the scalpel in

Sierra's chest. Not that I thought there would be any conscious retaliation; but I didn't want even a moment of irritation to distract from the business at hand.

Dr. Doyle said, "Look, we don't usually let parents be present in the catheterization. There's no need for it. The child is heavily sedated, doesn't feel anything and doesn't even remember anything. The parents, on the other hand, are not sedated, and they get upset. It distracts the technician and thereby endangers the patient."

"We understand that . . . that's why we wouldn't push it too much, but we've been advised that the catheterization is likely to be the scariest part of all for Sierra, just because she is sedated but not unconscious. The idea of her lying there, conscious, but powerless, watching strangers do something to her which is frightening, and being even more frightened by the feeling of having no power over her body or her mind . . . that seems a lot. If one of us were just sitting there, holding her hand, letting her know by our presence that everything is all right, we think that would be better."

Dr. Doyle was leaning back in her chair, listening. I couldn't tell if she was just being patient or whether she was actually interested. She said, "Mrs. Stoneman, we don't do these things unless it's for the well-being of the patient." We left it at that.

When I picked Sierra up at school that day, October 21st, her teacher told me Sierra had had her worst day ever. "We couldn't figure out what was wrong. She had several fights with other children that were unprovoked. She was very unlike herself."

"She knew we were going to see Dr. Doyle today. Maybe it had something to do with that," I replied, surprised that the tension was showing itself in this way.

We went to the Eighty-Second Street playground for a few hours and then home. While Sierra sat on her potty, I shared with her the results of our visit to Dr. Doyle. "Guess what, Sierra. We saw Dr. Doyle today and we decided not to have the operation until February."

"February? I don't want to have an operation anyway." This was the first time she had said she didn't want it.

"You don't want to have the operation at all?"

"No. I don't want an operation."

"Well, I can understand that. Have you been worrying about it?"

"Yes."

"Well, you don't need to worry about it for a while, because February is a long way off. You won't have the operation until after Halloween, after Thanksgiving, and after Christmas."

She was visibly relieved. Smiling broadly, laughing, she repeated, "After Halloween, after Thanksgiving, and after Christmas?"

"Right. And guess what else. Dr. Doyle said you wouldn't have to have any anal temperatures taken since you don't like that. She said she would write that on the record."

"She did!" Delighted, she giggled.

"Yup. We told her you didn't like those, so she said you didn't have to have any. And guess what else?

"What?" She was very open and interested now.

"She said at least one friend could come and visit you in the hospital."

"She did! Oh, good!" She laughed out loud again. "I want Annie to come. Can Annie come?"

"Sure it could be Annie. We had a really nice visit with Dr. Doyle. She told us everything that is going to happen."

We talked on a little about Dr. Doyle, then I said, "Guess what else, Sierra. I think I'm pregnant!"

"You are?" She was all excited. For the rest of the evening we had a long and intimate conversation about everything important. She asked me lots of questions about how babies are born, and how people make love, and how tiny she was when she was conceived, and where the eggs and sperm come from, and how people decide if they are going to have a baby. We lay on the bed together for a long time, talking, laughing, and sharing the way mothers and daughters dream of doing.

Sierra was used to John and me sharing whatever important things are going on. We thought if she's old enough to ask a question she's old enough to understand a simple answer. At least she's old enough to hear it, and later she can ask more questions if she doesn't understand. It's pretty much a toss-up who brings up something important. I might say, "Guess what, Sierra . . . " or she might say, "Mommy, I have something to say . . ."

For quite a while after this evening, none of us mentioned the operation. It was put off until after Christmas, so that was it.

In November we adopted a pretty white cat that had wandered into my office from the backyard and settled itself purring on my desk. In mid-December the cat disappeared. Sierra and I went up and down the block calling the cat, with no luck.

On the evening of December 18th the cat returned, filthy, dirty, and skinny. Sierra was very excited, more than I would have expected. I suggested we call someone up and tell them the cat was back. Sierra suggested Claude, Naveed's mother.

All halting and breathless, Sierra explained, "Guess what. This is some of my good news. The cat came back. Ana . . . who lives in my building . . . came home and first she didn't hear anything and then there was a cat noise . . . so she came in and told us and my mommy ran downstairs. We opened the door and went out and let the cat in. The cat was very dirty." Her speech was much less fluid than usual. She sounded as if she were two and a half, struggling to put sentences together. I wondered why.

She moved on, "You know why I'm lucky?" I expected her to say, "Because I got a lot of Christmas presents tonight and we put them under the tree." But no, she was working from a much deeper level on this phone call. She was plunged into telling Claude very important things about her life. "Because I have my own bed in the same room where my mommy and daddy sleep . . . and it has toys in it too already." Her voice was still breathless.

Intently, Sierra said to Claude, "Hold on a minute." She covered the phone with her hand, turned to me and said, "Am I going to have my operation after Christmas?"

"Yes."

She put the phone back to her mouth and said, "I'm going to have my operation after Christmas." I whispered, "In February," and she repeated that to Claude.

Just at that minute Claude was summoned off the phone by Naveed.

I was impressed and touched. "After Halloween, after Thanksgiving, and after Christmas," had been remembered! We hadn't mentioned the operation since that night in October. Sierra was evidently keeping track.

After talking with Claude, Sierra lay next to me in the bed. In very dramatic speech, with long pauses between each word, slapping my hand with hers on the enunciation of each word, Sierra said, "I . . . don't . . . want . . . to . . . have . . . my . . . I . . . V!" Anticipating the end, I joined her on the "V!" when our hands struck.

I picked it up, chanting, "I . . . can . . . understand . . . that . . . feeling." But I thought to myself, the IV will not be the worst this time. There will be worse. The catheterization will be worse. If she still has this fear of the IV, imagine what her recollection will be a year from now of all the worse things she's going to face.

Thinking we should get some of the fear of the IV released, I went on. "I wouldn't ... want to . . . have an . . . IV . . . either!"

She smiled. I said, "But . . . we . . . won't . . . have . . . any choice!" We were still slapping hands on each word. Then I got a little carried away, trying to help her express her fear. I said, "We . . . will . . . have . . . to . . . go . . . 'Aaaaah!'" I gave a little mock scream. Sierra said, "No!" with some anguish. I realized I had gone too far. Backing up, I said, "But remember how once you got the needle in your arm it didn't hurt at all, and you had to carry that big funny pole all over the place, even to the playroom?"

She bounced back, began to smile, and then laughed about the funny pole.

CHAPTER EIGHT

Mistakes

After Christmas we got moving. But we weren't free of anxiety. On December 28th my old friend David Kotz and his wife Karen came over. I hadn't seen David in a couple of years. In the interim they had adopted a baby because Karen had been sterilized by a fertility expert who had made several mistakes in treating an infection she had. They were involved in a malpractice suit.

"Oh God," we thought, "We don't even want to hear about doctors making mistakes. Serious life-threatening mistakes." The doctor involved had a perfectly good reputation. I was reminded of my friend whose father had died because he was given the wrong blood in a transfusion. Of course, this is really our biggest fear: MISTAKES. We know the statistics for the operation. We know it's not the most complicated operation. But MISTAKES get made even in simple procedures.

I decided to tackle the fear of mistakes directly. The next day I called Rodney. "Look Rodney. I want to know if I should be worrying about anything other than death for Sierra. That is, we've asked about the mortality statistics. Two percent doesn't sound so bad. But we haven't asked about the statistics for errors. What other things should we be worrying about?"

"You mean, mistakes like the little boy in Brooklyn who entered the hospital for a tonsillectomy and came out a vegetable?"

It was like a heavy thud in my gut. I hadn't heard about that little boy. "Yeah, that's what I mean. How can I find out about the mistake rate? The brain-damage rate?"

"Look," he said, "you can't find out. You have to trust. You have to say a lot of prayers, worry a lot, and trust. You have good doctors. Beyond that you should make sure you have a good anesthesiologist. Make sure he's Board certified, and tell him you're worried that they might not have the oxygen in the oxygen tanks so please check it."

"What! You mean I have to worry about that? You mean that could happen?"

"Yes. Things like that sometimes happen. When I was a third year resident, I always used to worry that they'd put the wrong gas in the tank."

Rodney's gift for telling me the truth but intruding his own anxieties into the situation struck again. I couldn't believe he had told me about children becoming vegetables, and oxygen tanks with the wrong gas. But at least he knew what I was talking about. He didn't pretend there was no such thing as mistakes. It reminded me that Olin, our psychiatrist friend, had told me the only reason for their keeping us out of the recovery room would be to make sure we didn't witness any mistakes, if any were made. My God. I guess the only thing to do is to trust the doctors, and make sure they're good.

The next day I asked my friend Doug Ades to ask his friend who had invented the bypass operation about Dr. Isom. He called back with the report, "Aces. Dr. Isom is an ace. Nothing to worry about."

I called a friend's pediatrician who worked at New York University Hospital. He said, "Dr. Doyle is the best. Dr. Isom is the one I'd choose myself. When my mother needed heart surgery last year it was Dr. Isom I chose, that's how highly I think of him. I'd trust him to operate on my own mother."

It's a good thing, I thought. Because he's operating on my own daughter.

Meanwhile John had found out from a friend who works there that New York University Hospital had a relatively high percentage of malpractice suits. He mercifully did not share this with me, knowing my fear of mistakes. He didn't think it was significant, because his source told him neither Dr. Isom nor Dr. Doyle were ever targets of these suits.

CHAPTER NINE

Sierra Decides

In January, one of our friends said, "Why are you putting Sierra through two hospitalizations if it could all be done in one? It sounds like she'll have to go through the preoperative experience twice, putting the IV in twice. If she's so scared, wouldn't it be better to do it only once?"

We had decided early on to have space of about two weeks between the two hospitalizations, so we could recuperate after one trauma before taking on another. But after our friend raised this question, it occurred to us that we had made this decision assuming it would be better for Sierra, without consulting Sierra. Of course, we had made all the decisions without consulting Sierra, without thinking twice about it. But she was getting older as time went on, and it now seemed that this decision was one she might have a strong opinion about.

John and I decided to consult Sierra. It was a little late, since the arrangements were already made; and we were actually still going on misinformation. We didn't even know yet that IVs would never be inserted except when Sierra was sedated.

Nonetheless, we waited for a leisurely dinner, and then I said, "We have a question to ask you Sierra. When you have your operation, first you have to have a test called a catheterization, which is almost like a little operation itself. We have a choice: either you can go to the hospital once, have the catheterization, come home for a week or so and go back for the real operation; or you can go into the hospital once and do it all at once."

"What kind of a test?" Sierra interrupted to ask.

"It's a test where they find out exactly where the narrow place is in your aorta."

"How do they do it?"

"They put a little needle into your leg by your crotch, and thread a little tiny tube up through your blood vessel close to your heart, and then they take pictures to see how your blood is moving. They can see where the blood gets stuck at the narrow place. Then they know exactly where it is."

"Will I feel it?"

"No."

"Will I be unconscious?"

"No, but you won't be aware of it. You'll have some medication to make sure you sleep."

"Oh."

"Anyway, do you think it would be better to do it all at once, the catheterization and the operation, or to have some time with us at home in between the test and the operation?" We held our breath, not knowing if we were pushing too far, asking her to think about it in this way.

After about a minute of silence, with Sierra in deep thought, she said firmly, "I think I should go two times and come home in the middle."

"Well, we're glad you think that. We think the same thing, so all of us have the same idea." Sierra looked very pleased, and maybe a little relieved that her judgment on such a big question had been corroborated by us. We explained that we thought it was a good idea to have time at home so everything wouldn't come all at once and she could rest in between.

We asked, "Would you like to know everything about the operation before it's going to happen?"

"Yes."

"Would you like to know way ahead of time or just a few days before?"

With strong feeling, Sierra asserted, "Start telling me way ahead. I can't learn it all so-fast, so-fast, so-fast, so-fast!" She shook her head back and forth on every, "so-fast," emphasizing what a whirl it would put her head into. I wondered what the strong feeling around "so fast" came from—was it the experience at Lenox Hill where things really did come too fast? Or was it an insight independent of any past negative experience? We were impressed that she knew so clearly what she wanted: preparation well in advance, and a rest in between the two procedures.

Soon after, Tim was having breakfast with us. He asked Sierra when she was going to have her operation. Since Tim had opened up the subject, I asked if she would like to visit the hospital today, with Naveed, to check out how it looks and how the playroom is. She looked nervous, and said no. She gave me an odd look, as if there were something suspicious going on. "You're going to be there with me all the time aren't you'?" The implication seemed to be that if I were going to be there she certainly didn't need to see the place ahead of time, so why the big deal about this one?

Then she added, "Except in the operation, right?"

Reluctantly, I said, "Right. And also not in the recovery room... and also not in the catheterization."

"Oh, yeah," she said, looking as if it took a little effort to absorb these reminders. "But you'll be there during the IV, right?"

"Right."

"But not in the cathet. . . catheter. . . catheterization?"

"Right."

She looked at me kind of wisely and brightly, and said, "Well, we'll see how that feels!"

Tim asked if she had met the doctor. She said, "No, but my parents have." She looked at me "Right?"

With some embarrassment I had to admit that we had not met the surgeon. I told her, "but we have met Dr. Doyle, and she's the one who's in charge of everything. We know the other doctor is very good also." But Sierra's tone of complete confidence that her parents had everything under control got under my skin. Of course, we should meet the surgeon. Sierra wants us to take care of everything, and not bother her with meeting too many doctors or visiting the hospital.

A few days later I called Dr. Doyle again. It was January 6th, and we were scheduled for February 9th.

"We're getting down to the wire. We are still thinking about the catheterization and the recovery room. I had the idea of proposing that one of us try being in a catheterization for another child to see if we could handle it, and then if we couldn't, no harm done, we'd just walk out. And if we could, maybe we could be there with Sierra."

"Mrs. Stoneman! This is getting to be more like managing the parents than the patient. This preoccupation with the catheterization is unhealthy. I don't approve of it, because the parents get upset and the technician gets distracted . . ."

"I know . . . that's the consideration we understand . . . that's why we haven't pushed it . . . but I want to let you know that's what's on our minds."

"I'll ask Dr. Danilowicz, but I don't favor it. You'd be more upset than Sierra. She'd be sedated, and you wouldn't. But maybe I can let you look at another 'cath' so you can see we're not torturing children."

"The thing is, Sierra is expressing a strong desire for us to be taking care of everything," I responded. "Sierra says

'You'll be with me all the time, right Mommy, except the operation?' And I have to say 'right, and the catheterization . . . and the recovery room . . . ' it begins to sound like a lot."

"Well," said Dr. Doyle, "the recovery room is no problem. You can be in there. As long as you don't become a problem, and then we'll put you right out."

I couldn't believe my ears! The big one. The recovery room! Just like that . . . "The recovery room is no problem." For months she had been saying we couldn't be in the recovery room. She jumped from our being a nuisance to yielding on the recovery room within two minutes. My head was spinning. I had tried to get through the conversation without alienating her, without sounding crazy, but still persisting . . . and Voila! A gift of the recovery room. I had no idea why.

"That's wonderful," I said in a mild understatement. "That makes a big difference. I think we're also ready to start meeting the other doctors at whatever pace you think is right. If we're not going to be in the 'cath' it may help to have some other familiar faces."

"I'll talk to Dr. Danilowicz." She sounded a little weary of the extra work we were laying on her. But I was elated. I called John right away and we both got very happy. Getting permission to be in the recovery room was important in itself. It had also taken on significance as proof that we were really doing our job as parents.

CHAPTER TEN

Final Preparations

THE NEXT MORNING SIERRA and I got into a major battle about her whining. It seemed she had been doing a lot of four-year-old whining lately, and I liked it less and less.

"Help me put on my tights," she said.

"OK, stand up so I can pull them up . . . "

"Nooooooooo . . . do it while I'm lying down."

That's how it began. The argument went on for twenty minutes. I refused to do it unless she stood up. She refused to stand up. This was what all our arguments boiled down to. A sheer test of wills. It had been the pattern since she was a tiny baby.

When I'd start to get annoyed, she'd say, "Don't talk mad at me!" And I'd say "Well, don't whine at me." She'd end up screaming at the top of her very strong lungs. Often, I gave in. But that morning I didn't . . . that's why it lasted so long. She finally stood up.

Whenever these battles occurred, I would start to worry about Sierra's ability to handle the operation. If she couldn't stand not having everything as she likes it, how would she be able to stand an operation with all the pain and inconvenience?

After the struggle I drove her to school, along our usual route down the West Side Highway. The pretty Hudson River was covered with ice; the sky was bright blue. We were both lost in our thoughts, in that calm that follows any battle in which I have refused to give in. She was subdued. I was wondering if she was thinking about the operation these days. I wondered if her worry could be contributing to these fights.

At that moment, Sierra said, "When I have my operation, will I be unconscious during the IV?" My wondering was answered. "No, you'll be awake."

"No, Daddy told me I'd be unconscious."

"Then we'd better talk with John, because I don't think that's right. I think they use the IV to put into your body the medicine that makes you unconscious, so they have to put the IV in first." In fact, I was wrong about this. We still had not gotten a blow-by-blow description of what would happen during the operation.

"Oh," Sierra said. "Annie had a hernia. What's a hernia?"

"A torn muscle that has to be sewn back up."

'That's what Annie had. The same thing as me. An operation. She was only three."

"I think she was even younger . . . , maybe even two," I said.

"How was it? How did Annie feel about it?" Sierra asked.

"I think the part she didn't like was when the doctor made her take an anal temperature."

"Yeah. In her anus."

"Are you starting to think about the operation a little?" I asked.

"Yes, I'm starting to feel a little scared about it." That was straightforward, I thought.

"Would you like us to tell you everything that's going to happen? Exactly what's going to happen when you go in the hospital'?"

"Yes," Sierra said without any hesitation.

"OK. Tonight, John and I will get our notes from our meeting with the doctor and we'll tell you exactly what will happen."

"Can you tell me exactly?"

"Well, almost exactly. There are always a few surprises . . . like a different nurse comes and does it a different way, or a doctor changes a decision . . . but almost exactly we can tell you."

"OK," she said calmly. Almost exactly seemed good enough.

"Do you want to start visiting the doctors?"

"No. You go to the doctors and tell me what they say."

We reached Calhoun School and I parked the car. Sierra climbed onto my lap and put her arms tightly around my neck. I carried her up the stairs to school, feeling very close to her. Whenever she really tells me how she feels she seems so very vulnerable. She was working really hard at all of this.

The next day Dr. Doyle called me back. "Mrs. Stoneman, it's arranged for one of you to meet with Dr. Danilowicz and see a catheterization. But I hope you're doing this for the welfare of the patient, not for your own interest."

"Dr Doyle," I responded, "I don't understand your suspicions. Why else would we be doing it?"

"Well," she said, "Frankly, I'm always suspicious of writers. They have a way of using this for the trade."

"Then I'll send my husband."

"All right. He should meet Dr. Danilowicz at nine a.m. on Wednesday."

I was surprised that Dr. Doyle was suspicious of me. I never considered myself a writer; but, of course, I had sent her the only two articles I'd ever had published, and they were about Sierra and the doctors. I decided I had better not tell her until this was all over that I was indeed keeping some notes of our experience and planning to write something. My motive was to give myself some perspective and help other parents and children, but she seemed to be assuming there would be an opportunist element, so I didn't want to expose myself to more distrust. I remembered that when I first wrote the little article about Rodney and Sierra, I didn't show it to him for a couple of years. When I did, he was very enthusiastic, convinced I should send it to Dr. Doyle and should write more for parents. Maybe Dr. Doyle would similarly find it useful afterwards.

John went to meet with Dr. Danilowicz. As it turned out, she didn't let him see an actual catheterization, but she showed him the room and the equipment and went over the whole procedure detail by detail.

We have found when dealing with doctors it is always good to ask everyone involved to tell you the whole story, because each one provides a few details that the others left out. Finally, it becomes possible to piece together a more complete story. Furthermore, if the doctors disagree with each other, it's possible to pursue the question until they agree.

This was no exception. Dr. Danilowicz told John that if they failed to get through the aorta coming up through the artery from the groin, they would then make an incision in her right arm and go up through that artery. This was new information.

She also showed him a special table onto which they strap the patient. This table rolls back and forth, allowing the x-ray camera to take pictures of the patient's whole chest. This information became an important part of Sierra's preparation.

The next week, the week of February 1st, John spent several evenings with Sierra in which he took her through every step of the catheterization. He has a genius for playing with children, making things funny. By the time I got home from a class one evening, the two of them were full of laughter about the rolling bed, and the turning bed, and strapping her onto it. She was very happy and very close to John. It seemed that he had relieved her anxieties with his conversation and his play. They had acted out the whole thing.

On Tuesday and Wednesday the week before the catheterization, John and Sierra kept playing out the sequence of the catheterization, with as many jokes and as much laughter as John could create.

By this time John and I were back to looking at the cardiology books. One of them was a wonderful big picture book which had page after page of colored pictures of every kind of heart operation. Sierra found this one fascinating too. By now she had seen many, many, pictures of a coarctation. We figured that she would give us an indication if we were pushing too much information on her. But the books interested her a lot, with no apparent anxiety attached.

On Thursday our friend Stella Saltonstall took Sierra and me out to lunch at a fancy restaurant and took Sierra to buy a pretty dress. Stella made no mention of the connection between this event and Sierra's operation. She wanted Sierra to have the feeling that she didn't have to be sick or in the hospital to get presents. But I suspected that Sierra was quite clear about the reason people were starting to give her presents. Saturday evening when she and I were cooking together, I started to say, "If you . . . " and stopped. Sierra picked it right up, "If I what?" I reluctantly finished my thought, "If you could have any three presents you wanted, what would they be?"

Sierra said, "You mean for my operation? I want lipstick."

On Friday afternoon we picked Sierra up early from school to go see Dr. Doyle for a routine checkup before hospitalization. The five-year-olds in her class at school wanted to know why Sierra needed an operation, so I sat in their circle and explained, "Sierra has a very narrow place in the big blood vessel that takes blood from her heart to the rest of her body. The blood is having trouble getting through that narrow place, so the doctors are going to take out the narrow place and sew the ends together so the blood can go through."

Immediately all the five-year-olds began telling of their experiences with doctors and hospitals. There seemed to be a craving to discuss them. Sierra stood nearby, listening, apparently very comfortable with the attention from everybody.

Other parents later told us their children had been very worried about Sierra because she had graphically explained everything that was going to happen to her in several different school discussions. While she seemed to have integrated the idea of doctors cutting into her body, reaching inside and fixing things, enough to explain it all in detail and without upset, the other children found it a little scary. Her friend Elizabeth didn't sleep the night Sierra was supposed to go to the hospital.

As we drove from school to Dr. Doyle's office, I suggested that after the operation I could come back to her own class of five-year-olds to explain everything to them. Sierra said, "Yes, because you will still be out of work." It is important to her that I have taken this time off from work to be with her. But I thought I had better warn her that it wouldn't go on forever. "Well, soon after the operation I will be going back to work."

Sadly, she asked, "WHY?"

"Because you'll be going back to school to be with your friends, so I'll go back to work where I can do good things for people and make some money to pay for our dinners.

"For our dinners? What do you mean?"

"Well," I said lamely, "the money has to come from somewhere to buy food, so I have to work." Perhaps I felt I wasn't supposed to love my work so much, so I used the same excuse men have used for generations.

John asked Sierra if she had any questions for Dr. Doyle. "I have one question," Sierra replied, "but it's a secret. I'll ask it myself."

We stopped to buy some green beans and some apple juice, and we crunched on them as we walked toward Bellevue. Then we skipped, and laughed, and made some jokes. These trips to the hospital were always special. All three of us were always together, and John and I were always on our best, most loving behavior, because the awareness of what was coming was uppermost in our minds. Sierra walked along the stone walls holding my hand, drinking her juice. We skipped down the ramp to Bellevue, laughing and holding hands. People stepped to the side, smiling. One person commented, "Somebody's happy!"

This was only the third time Sierra had ever seen Dr. Doyle. It was still a special event. Sierra sat with shy anticipation on my lap, alert to everything. She reached for the heart model to look at it up close. John and I sat back with foolish little grins on our faces while Dr. Doyle talked to Sierra in a very lovely way. Sierra obviously liked her.

I asked Sierra if she wanted to ask her a question. She whispered back, "You ask it. I want to know if I'll be having IV."

"Sierra wants to know if she'll be having an IV."

"You'll get an IV before surgery, but it will be after they give you the medication that will make you very sleepy, so you won't feel much of any pain."

We began to ask our other questions: "Will Sierra feel much pain after the surgery?"

"Can't we wait for these questions until after the catherization?" Dr. Doyle asked.

"We could, but we're getting questions now that we'd like to be able to answer."

Sierra will have some pain," Dr. Doyle explained, "but not as much as grown-ups would feel. Children get over these things so quickly. She'll have a little pain for a day or two." Sierra was heard to repeat this several times. She loved it that children don't feel as much pain as adults.

We went into the examining room, where Sierra seemed almost elated. I wished I could take pictures of the examination, because the happy look on Sierra's face, coupled with the caring look on Dr. Doyle's face, would have made a great advertisement for pediatrics. There was some magical quality about the interaction between them every time.

Dr. Doyle introduced us to the technicians who were to do the echogram. An echogram sends sound waves that bounce off the heart; they create a picture of the heart beating. Sierra was fitted with electrodes, asked to lie down, and then a little pencil-like buzzing instrument was held against her chest for about twenty minutes. John and I stood arm in arm watching the film, listening to the two discussing it.

"See, it occasionally moves into five chambers . . . see the flopping of the valve . . . " These phrases caught my fearful ear. Five chambers? Flopping valve? It didn't sound right. I felt a catch in my throat as I remembered that the purpose of all these tests was to find out if Sierra had any more anomalies in addition to the coarctation.

We watched while they recorded onto the videotape, "This is the tape of Sierra Stoneman-Bell," and I wondered if they ever mixed up the tapes, giving the doctor the wrong one. That must be why they stated the name of the patient on the videotape itself; they didn't just write it on the outside of the container. I wondered if we were watching competent technicians or ones that somebody had already decided needed to be fired because they had revealed incompetence. Surely people must get fired from hospital staffs—that means they are here right up until the day they're fired. Surely there are people we will meet who are on the verge of being fired.

They were very friendly and kind technicians, who gladly played the film back for Sierra. I asked my questions, timidly, about what the five chambers and the flopping valve meant. They laughed and assured me it was perfectly normal. We had asked Dr. Doyle if she could give us an empty IV bottle for Sierra to play with. Just as we finished the echogram she returned with a full set, and whispered conspiratorially, "I suggest you bury it in your pocketbook . . . I don't know if they'll stop you at the doors, but bury it deep." The technicians also gave us a handful of round electrodes that could be stuck to the body. Sierra was delighted with all her loot.

"They're not fake!" she bragged. "I have an IV set and lots of other hospital stuff and it's not fake!"

That evening I was eager to play with the IV set, but Sierra deliberately ignored it. We ended up watching television late into the evening. *The Incredible Hulk* and *Dallas* were Sierra's choices of entertainment. We have an agreement that we will change the channel whenever things get bad for children—violent or scary. We have always encouraged her to hide her eyes if something scary comes on without warning, but this night she was determined to watch everything scary, eyes wide open.

On the way out of the hospital that afternoon Sierra had gotten it into her head that she wanted a big chocolate Easter egg with a shiny wrapper. I said, "No." We had decided not to yield on TV and candy during this period. I had a big urge to let her have all the candy she wanted, to give her everything; but that would be very suspicious to her, and very foolish of me. So, I said no, and she had a huge tantrum in the hospital anteroom.

That night the issue came up again: candy for dessert although she'd already had her sweets quota for the day. I continued to say no, and allowed her to have another tantrum. It occurred to me that she was using the candy issue to relieve some general tension, so I encouraged her to have it out, being very loving and patient and not getting angry even when she tried to kick me. Her friend Quiana was there, quite impressed with this freedom to have a tantrum; so she started to climb into my lap and cry too.

Sierra said, "Get off her lap. I want to sit there." They started to push each other. Finally, Sierra welcomed Quiana, pulling her into her arms. I said, "Quiana loves you." Sierra said, "I love her too and of course I love you because you're my mother." I said, "I love you and we all love each other . . . " Finally we were all piled on top of each other laughing on the kitchen floor professing undying love for each other, the tantrums having been transformed into loving intimacy.

That night when we went to bed, Sierra and John and I lay together for a while. She said, "Some parents are mean, aren't they? Bryan's parents spank him. Some parents in the supermarket talk so mean and fast to their children.

What does *scold* mean and what does *punish* mean? Why do some parents threaten their children?"

We tried our best to answer the questions, and told her how punishments used to be really bad. We told her about the stocks they used in Puritan days.

"What don't you believe in?"

"Do you mean . . . we don't believe in spanking?"

"That's what I meant," she said. Then she asked if Bryan's parents would spank her if she did something bad. Answering her own question, she said, "No, they wouldn't, because you wouldn't let them."

Her enormous trust that we would protect her from harm triggered a new obsession for me. I began to visualize her after the operation, victim of oxygen shortage, looking up at me with a damaged brain and an expression on her face that asked implicitly, "How could you have let this happen to me?"

After all, I thought, we've told her everything about the operation except there are risks attached. Do we have the right to take her life into our hands in this way without her permission? If she knew what we knew, that the risks are small compared to the near certainty of hemorrhaging and early death without the operation, she would undoubtedly choose what we have chosen. But she hasn't had that choice. This idea bothered me enough that I called Harvey Jackins, the founder of Re-evaluation Counseling, and laid it out, asking advice. He assured me that we were doing the right thing, and the idea of sharing the decision with

Sierra was just an effort to relieve my own anticipated guilt in case something went wrong. Keep my anxiety and guilt to myself, he advised, and be confident that Sierra will always be grateful that we had the courage to decide on an operation even though she had no visible symptoms. But an analysis of the risks is our business as adults, not hers.

This would seem obvious to most people. But then, most people wouldn't consult their four-year-old on whether to go to the hospital once or to go twice with a rest in between. I knew our respect for Sierra's intelligence is usually right, and I knew that Harvey approved of it. So, his clarity on the question of sharing the risks relieved me of that question.

On Saturday morning, February 7th, we started playing with the IV set. Sierra said she would be the nurse, John would be the doctor, and I would be the patient. John insisted that she be the doctor, because he is a convinced women's liberationist. They finally compromised and agreed that they both could be doctors.

As the doctor, Sierra showed an extreme desire not to hurt me. She inserted the IV so carefully, not even wanting to get it close to my skin, just taping it on my hand with gauze. I got kind of interested in actually poking my finger with a finger stick to put real blood into our test tubes, but she wouldn't hear of it. She just followed me around with the IV, holding it out for me while I did other things.

In the middle of the game John went off to do some desk work. Shortly after that I went to sleep on the dining room floor. When I woke up, I just wanted to cry about how they had better not kill her. Both John and I were irritable and began to argue about why he stopped playing with us and why I went to sleep.

All day Saturday we kept snapping at each other. Finally, after Sierra went to sleep, we had a major fight, revealing that both of us were really upset. The fight brought us good relief, because I was somehow able to swing into being a counselor, encouraging John to get really mad at me. This time my having enough slack to encourage and absorb his anger and apologize for my irritability broke the tension and we ended the evening at two a.m. feeling very close.

On Sunday, Sierra was so excited and happy about going to the hospital the next day that it reminded me of her birthday party. I couldn't detect any signs of fear. She was showing complete trust in us, an interest in all that was going to happen, and she was hyped up like before Christmas.

She came to me at breakfast and started tying the IV around my hand again. Again, I was the patient, not her. John was the father. We went all through the operation with Sierra again representing the soft line all the way. Every time I wanted something she gave it to me. When I wanted to eat, even before the operation, she let me. When I wanted to drink, even in the recovery room, she let me. I was allowed to have all the ice cream I wanted. I asked, "Can I have some candy, doctor?" "Well," she said, "Because it's a special treat, since you had an operation . . . you can have . . . (long deep pause) . . . three candies."

Our role seemed delicate. How much should we play it her way? How much should we give information as we go along? I decided to give information by acting uncomfortable and in pain at those points where I thought she would be feeling it. It seemed to surprise her a little, and she moved to eliminate the pain each time.

I had Sierra read out loud to me in her role as a doctor. Her reading had taken a leap forward, and I liked building it into the game. She read thirty-six pages of her little primer to me, very proudly. I felt pleased that we were not just single-mindedly focusing on the operation, but that we were helping her learn other things too.

At dinner I asked Sierra if we should take the time to tell our guests, Tom and Tim, everything that was going to happen. She said, "You," with enjoyment. So, I ran upstairs and brought down my notes. I began telling Tom and Tim, step by step. Sierra interjected what she knew. It was perfect. Together, the five of us went over everything. A lot of laughing, because John did half of it and made it funny—especially the part about the rolling bed and her being strapped in during the catheterization.

I said, "In the evening tomorrow the nurses will come to take your pulse and temperature . . . (we stopped to take all our pulses, because she didn't know what that was) . . . but remember Dr. Doyle said no anal temperature because you don't like that . . . but still, probably some nurse will come to do it and I'll say, 'Dr. Doyle gave her permission not to have it anally,' and the nurse will say, 'Dr. Doyle didn't say anything,' and I'll say, 'She did promise us, go and look on the record,' and the nurse will look and she'll come back and say, 'It's not on the record' and I'll say, 'call her up, she did say it' until finally she'll give up. Things like that might happen." Sierra told me to tell the story about when I was hiding under the bed at Lenox Hill Hospital. So I did. We all laughed a lot.

Something came up about an enema. Sierra said she didn't know what that was. I reminded her she'd had several in Lenox Hill. She said she hadn't cried. I laughed and said she had screamed her head off. She laughed and laughed. She said, "That's impossible or I wouldn't have a head." I said she had screamed and yelled, and she was very smart because while she screamed she yelled instructions to the nurses: "Count to ten so I'll know when it's going to be over."

She volunteered that the reason she couldn't eat anything between midnight and the morning was that the medication for sleep might give her an upset stomach. We laughed about how they would wake her up in the morning to give her a shot to put her to sleep. She volunteered that the shot would hurt, but only for a minute. This whole recounting took a full half hour in which Tom and Tim gave very full attention. It was a perfect way to do it.

CHAPTER ELEVEN

The Roller Coaster

FEBRUARY 9, 1981. IT was finally here.

Our little bags were packed. The sun was shining on a cold clear winter day. While I was dressing Sierra she remarked, "I think it's going to be fun in the hospital." I seized on this as my opportunity to give her the little warning that had been percolating in my mind: "Yes, it probably will be fun. But don't be surprised if there are some scary times and some hard times too."

With my encouragement, Sierra herself called the hospital to confirm that they had a bed ready. "This is Sierra Stoneman-Bell. Do you have a bed ready for me today?"

The receptionist hung up. She undoubtedly thought it was a prank. I called back.

"I'm sorry Mrs. Stoneman-Bell. There is no bed free for Sierra today. You will have to call again tomorrow. Yes, we know she is scheduled to be admitted today, but these things are not always predictable."

My heart sank. Surprise number one. We were all ready, but the hospital wasn't.

We valiantly changed gears and I took Sierra off to school, making exciting plans all the way: she would read her primer to her teachers, we would invite her teachers to dinner, we would get a fried chicken for lunch, I would stay and take pictures of all her friends. We had a whole exciting day set up, and her teachers had agreed to it, when suddenly one of her teachers ran out to where we were eating our fried chicken in front of the school. "Call home," she said. "They do have a bed for you, after all."

Suddenly I was upset. Sierra and I had made other plans. We were not ready any more. They had no right to confuse us like this.

With a quiver in her voice, Sierra said, "I don't want to go to the hospital."

"I know how you feel, Sierra. This is one of those surprises we talked about. But it's not right. They got us all mixed up. First no bed, now a bed, after we had made other plans. Now we're all mixed up. But I refuse to rush. We're eating our chicken first, with your friends."

As we drove home to get John, Sierra said, "You're the best Mommy in the whole world . . .Well . . . not the best in the world, because I haven't met the other Mommies. But you're the best woman I have." She was struggling with her idea that it's not nice to say anyone is best. I don't know where she got this strong idea. I tried to temper it slightly, saying, "Well, you're the best daughter in the world to me. To me you're very special, because I'm your Mommy."

"OK," she replied, "but you shouldn't tell me that in front of any other kids. It might hurt their feelings."

"All right, but I will tell you when we're alone."

"And I won't tell them that you said it," she said conspiratorially.

Finally, all three of us were zooming down the East River Drive, Sierra on my lap clutching the doll Stella had bought for her, and John at the wheel. We were heading for New York University Hospital, where a bed was ready for Sierra.

From the car to the hospital Sierra sang little songs to herself, and talked to her doll. We couldn't catch the words. In the waiting room she and John played actively throughout our hour-and-a-half wait. They ran, and read, and colored. Another little four-and-a-half-year-old appeared and we purposefully befriended her to continue peer support on the ward.

Surprise number two: the hospital put us on the East Ward with teenagers instead of on the West Ward with small children. John was mildly annoyed, because he had already met the nursing staff on the West Ward and had liked them.

As we walked tentatively onto the ward a little child came zooming toward us on a scooter. "Oh," I thought to myself, "Good. A healthy child having a lot of fun. This is a good greeting for Sierra." but as he approached, we were all simultaneously struck by the little boy's alarming appearance. His hair had been shaved and he had great big stitches running from one ear over the top of his head to the other ear, in wavy lines. It looked like the two halves of his head had been sewn together. One of his eyes had stitches on the lid, making it look sewn shut. John and I looked at each other, big eyed, remembering that Dr. Doyle had warned us. "Remember when Dr. Doyle told us we would see some strange-looking people getting problems fixed?" one of us said quickly as we hurried to the protective cover of our room.

Safely inside, Sierra did not want to venture back out on the ward. When I suggested we go explore, she said, "No, I don't want to see any more strange-looking people." We agreed that I would go on a scouting expedition.

After a thorough tour of the ward, I was able to report that the strangest looking person was the one we had already seen, and that he did not seem so strange when I talked to him in the playroom.

For the rest of the afternoon we played with the wonderful bed that went up and down at the top, the bottom, and in the middle. We waited for the myriad admissions procedures that took from three to nine p.m. One after another, different ward personnel came in to ask us questions. In very serious tones they asked about symptoms and history.

Over and over we had to say, "No, she's never had any symptoms. No, no getting blue, no clubbing, no heavy nosebleeds, no nothing." It began to seem crazy that we were in the hospital with this perfectly healthy child preparing for major surgery answering questions from overly serious trainees of various levels. Sierra began to feel weird.

She climbed into my arms, tucked her own arms under her belly, trying to be as close to me as possible.

I sensed her feeling. "Too many people asking the same questions in a very serious way, right? Acting like it's a big deal."

"Right," she said.

But when we went to get the x-rays taken it was sheer enjoyment. Sierra loved the big machine. She climbed up onto a box, and into a kind of capsule that the technician made rise by pressing a button. He was very jolly and friendly, and she loved it. The technician said he wished all the children were like Sierra. The people in the waiting room were smiling at her. A one-legged sour-pussed man we'd seen in admissions was there; even he smiled at Sierra. There was a circle of people waiting in chairs, with Sierra in the middle practicing skipping.

"Look, Mommy."

"I am," I said. "In fact, we all are!" All the people smiled and began to converse with us. It was a nice few minutes, breaking the somewhat depressed mood of a group of isolated noncommunicating people, most of whom were dreading their own surgery.

All afternoon Sierra had been fearfully anticipating the finger prick. This was expected to be the one hurting thing of the day, but the hours ticked by until evening. Finally, the finger-pricking lady with a tray of blood tubes and a rapid flow of reassuring words arrived. She plunked down her tray, whipped out a finger-pricking machine and said, "Give me a finger."

Sierra said, "No, that's too fast."

The woman said, "Give me your finger. You won't feel a thing. It's over in a second. See?" And she held up the finger-pricking machine and snapped it closed. It looked sinister—a hard snapping thing.

"Why do you do it so hard?" Sierra asked.

"Not so hard," she said, "Watch while I do it to the doctor." She snapped it on the finger of a nearby doctor. Sierra decided to take a chance. She stuck out her finger, the lady snapped the machine on her finger and hardly a ripple crossed Sierra's face. "Is this all?" she said.

We called this surprise number three, because we thought it would hurt and it didn't. Sierra was happy for the rest of the night.

In the evening one procedure was for John to sign a consent to the catheterization. Dr. Danilowicz had warned him that the consent form was frightening because they had only one form that they used for all patients, and the scary parts really only applied to old people and sick infants. She said to disregard paragraph two.

When John received it, he was prepared to ignore this terrible paragraph. But he showed it to me, and it seared itself into my mind: "I understand that the catheterization can cause death, paralysis, arrhythmia, loss of the use of one arm . . . " There were about seven lines of equally frightening things. The next paragraph said, "I do not want further information about these risks."

I didn't sign it. I didn't feel right about a doctor warning us that we should ignore that paragraph. If it were important enough to put on the consent form it was important enough to understand fully. If it didn't apply to us, they should give us a different consent form. But John was the one who had visited the catheterization lab and talked with the doctor, so I trusted his judgment.

That evening the nurse, Vinnie, was supposed to get Sierra's blood pressure. But he couldn't get it; there was evidently not enough pressure in her legs to measure. He went up the hierarchy: first Vinnie, then the student doctor, then another nurse, then the resident in charge, then a special machine and blood pressure technician. But the special machine didn't work properly so they had to try over and over again, on Sierra's legs especially. Sierra held a long, animated conversation with our friend John D'Emilio while the hospital staff went through this parade, exclaiming repeatedly how patient and cooperative she was. Other children, they said, would be having a fit by now. But in her wise way, Sierra responded, "I don't see any point in having a struggle. It only hurts a little."

The big hurt was scheduled for the morning: two shots. John and I both stayed overnight, sleeping fitfully, while Sierra enjoyed a sound sleep.

The nurses came on schedule at 7:30 a.m. with two needles: Thorazine and Demerol, and something else. I later learned the something else was designed to give Sierra amnesia, to prevent nightmares after the procedure. The medications couldn't be mixed so two needles were necessary.

Amazingly, Sierra went through these long-expected shots with ease. She let them do it after the slightest delay and two or three whimpers. She watched them insert the needles in her leg, and instead of holding on tight to my body as she would have the year before, she sat on my lap and merely clung to my fingers. During the insertion of the syringe, which went deep and was held there, she let out one deep wail, but still let them do it, crying only very briefly afterwards. John and I were impressed. Sierra was proud. We had no reason to suspect there would be a severe crisis later involving Sierra's reaction to shots.

Within half an hour she began to nod out. When the nurse came with the "rolling bed," Sierra went on it easily, rousing herself for only a second to say with urgent grogginess, "My pillow." We walked alongside the bed to the elevator as promised by Dr. Danilowicz. At the elevator a lady stopped us.

"You're not allowed on this elevator."

"But we were promised that we could walk down with her."

"Well. You'll have to take the other elevator then."

"Do you promise that someone else won't meet us down there and say we're not allowed on the sixth floor?"

"I don't know, but you can't come on this elevator."

"OK, we'll meet you on the sixth floor."

We ran and caught the other elevator. Emerging from it, we caught sight of Sierra being wheeled down the corridor and around the corner away from us. The lady was certainly not waiting for us for one second. We ran to catch up. Sierra was quite out. Another young woman who introduced herself as Maureen was waiting to receive her at the door.

"Will you please explain to Sierra what's going on, even though she seems to be asleep? We believe it makes some impression on her anyway, and she can hear what's going on."

"Of course," said Maureen, in a classically reassuring way. "I'll take good care of her." At that point Sierra roused herself again, and said, "My pillow!" We chuckled, having expected her to say "No, don't go!" We said a quick goodbye to Sierra and left for the elevator.

While Sierra was downstairs, we ate breakfast and hugged and cried and talked a lot. John and I had been edgy with each other, but edging closer to each other through this. We both wanted to heal the distance in our relationship at the same time as Sierra's heart was getting healed. Our lack of time together over the past few years of my work escalation had begun to show irritable rifts and a kind of numb distance that scared me. My decision to spend two full months attending to Sierra was encouraged by knowing that John and I needed some time too, for all our sakes.

We finally got word, at 10 a.m., that Sierra had handled everything fine and would be coming up in twenty minutes.

"Here she comes," someone said. They wheeled Sierra in. It was a precious moment. I reached into the bed to help move her on to her own bed, and she roused herself with bleary eyes to say, "Lie down on the bed with me." So I lay down with her in my arms. Her face was very pale, her lips very dry. She looked very fragile. John lay down with us.

I don't know how long we lay there, together, peacefully, on the bed with the sun pouring in the big window and the skyscrapers visible in the distance. Maybe about half an hour.

Then the crisis began, when the nurse came to take Sierra's pulse and could not find it in Sierra's right arm. It had been necessary to go through the artery in her arm, because the coarctation prevented the catheter from passing through from the groin to the heart. As a result, Sierra did have three stitches in her right arm. The nurse also noticed that her right hand was chilly.

This was a young nurse, not experienced with reassuring parents, so when I asked her what that could mean she said, "A cold hand is one of the things we look for after a cath. It could mean they didn't stitch up her arm properly."

Oh, God. Here it is. The mistake. I held off my alarmist reaction, and said, "Would you please check it out?" Actually, my memory isn't too clear here, but I felt the blood rushing to my head, felt the fear rising. Her hand was cold. There was no pulse. Did that mean hemorrhage? Was she bleeding inside? Was she in danger? Would she lose the use of one arm?

Within minutes . . . it seemed longer . . . the resident doctor came. She said, "I'm actually not too worried about it. This happens. The artery goes into spasm and temporarily the blood doesn't pass through so well. But I'll page Dr. Danilowicz."

She wasn't too worried . . . but she was worried enough to page a doctor.

There was nothing for us to do but wait. We lay there with Sierra, looking at each other, absorbed in a silent panic.

Dr. Danilowicz did not answer the page. An agonizing half an hour passed. Finally, Dr. Doyle arrived, cool and colorful, with a bright orange dress under her doctor's white coat, and bright orange lipstick under her tinted yellow hair. She smiled, seeing us all in bed together and said, "The whole family." She reached down for Sierra's hand, felt for the pulse, pinched the flesh on her fingers and hand, compared the temperature between the two hands and said, "Her pulse is weak. Her hand is a little cool. Her circulation is good. Often the artery will have a little spasm after the cath, but it will open out again. This is not unusual. But we'll watch it. Don't worry about it."

Our panic drained away, and a composed relief took its place as Dr. Doyle delivered the initial findings on the catheterization to us. She stood, dignified and warm and distant, on the other side of our little cubby hole, and said, "The initial results of the catheterization show that Sierra has a discrete coarctation in the usual place with no other abnormalities in the heart valves. The coarctation is very severe, very severe. The catheter could not get past it coming up from her groin. But there are no other complications. I haven't looked at all the pictures yet, but these are the preliminary findings."

With a word of reminder that Sierra might feel sick to her stomach this afternoon, she left.

Just as John and I turned to each other to share our relief from the panic about the arm, Sierra sat up and began to vomit. We expected that. Vomiting was fine. But what came bursting out of her mouth when she wretched was nothing but blood. Dark brownish blood.

I leapt off the bed and out into the corridor. "Dr. Doyle! . . . Nurse . . . Sierra's vomiting blood . . . get Dr. Doyle." The nurse ran behind me, and then swerved back to get Dr. Doyle on another ward. Within minutes Dr. Doyle again strode calmly in, all orange and yellow and white. She surveyed the scene of John and me in a panic, blood all over the bed clothes, and she said, "Did Sierra have a bloody nose last night?"

"Yes."

"Well, that's it. She swallowed some of the blood and that's what's coming up now." She smiled at us, "Sierra won't develop an acute ulcer that quickly . . . YOU might."

When she left, John and I laughed and laughed. I lay back down with Sierra in my arms, and John sat there making mock terrified faces, while we both laughed and laughed. He imitated a panic-stricken person rushing for help, motioning frantically with his hands and twisting his face all up in exaggerated fear, and we laughed. God, what a roller coaster of emotions.

It took the afternoon to recover from the giddy feeling that we'd been through a wringer. We shared it with all our visitors, while Sierra slept on.

Doctors still came in and out, checking Sierra's hand. On a later visit Dr. Doyle said, "If it doesn't warm up, we'll have the surgeon take a look at it and maybe give it some heparin." Oh, blood clots. I knew enough to know heparin was an anticoagulant. But blood clots mean rushing to the brain and causing strokes . . . isn't that an emergency? But they weren't treating it as an emergency. Next morning both Dr. Danilowicz and Dr. Doyle said she was fine and could go home.

When we got home our friend John D'Emilio was waiting there to play with Sierra so John and I could relax together. This was part of the program of the Sierra Stoneman-Bell Heart Club, which our friend Judy Ennes had organized months before. Our personal friends and members of the Re-evaluation Counseling Community in New York had joined together to make sure that John, Sierra, and I all had adequate support to make it through.

Forty-three people were in the Heart Club. All of them visited and offered co-counseling attention to us in and out of the hospital, during the three hospitalizations that turned out to be necessary. Some of them played with Sierra so John and I could be with each other. Some of them counseled each of us individually so we could give our best to Sierra. This extraordinary show of skilled and loving support meant the world to us. It qualitatively changed the experience from a life crisis handled by a little knot of three people bound together in a nuclear family beset with irrational anxieties and emotional and physical exhaustion, to a wondrous experience of an ad hoc community rallying itself together on behalf of members facing a crisis. We are forever grateful to all our friends and counselors who came through for us in this generous and thoughtful way.

The next two weeks passed quickly. Sierra seemed delighted with herself. She had no nightmares and no apparent dread of the return to the hospital. Her hand gradually recovered its full warmth and full use, under our watchful eyes.

John and I, on the other hand, had a plethora of nightmares. One night we were both awake for four hours, tossing and turning, talking and crying, interspersed with nightmares about fighting Hitler and swarms of rats.

The next morning we called Dr. Doyle for sheer reassurance. We asked her about Dr. Isom: how many coarc operations has he done, why she thought it would work out well, had there ever been any bad results . . .

She assured us that he'd done over sixty coarcs, with never a bad result of any kind: never a repeat operation to correct anything. She assured us that the anesthesiologists were excellent and all board certified. "Everything's going to be good," she said. We had learned to believe her.

During these weeks we kept our long-scheduled appointment to meet Dr. Isom. He turned out to be a friendly, large, fortyish man with a heavy southern drawl, followed everywhere by a retinue of resident surgeons who did everything he did immediately after he did it. When Dr. Isom listened to Sierra's heart, his followers lined up and listened in turn. When he looked in her ears, his followers did the same. When he sat behind his desk for a conversation, his court stood in a row and listened to every word. He must be very good, we thought.

While we were talking with Dr. Isom, Sierra leaned over and whispered in my ear, "Mommy, why doesn't he have a thumb?"

Directing my eyes to his right hand, I saw, sure enough, the right-handed surgeon was lacking a thumb.

"Dr. Isom," I said casually, "Sierra would like to know why you don't have a thumb." It's always useful to attribute curiosity to the child.

"Well," he chuckled, "you're very observant, Sierra. I don't have a thumb because when I was a little boy about five years old I got my thumb accidentally in the way of my mother's hedge clippers when she was clipping a hedge."

Theoretically a thumbless surgeon would be just the thing to make us nervous. But it didn't. He had built his reputation on excellence, not on his thumb. It was simply amazing.

CHAPTER TWELVE

The Crisis

On our way to New York University Hospital on March 4th for the surgery, we had to stop off at Bellevue Hospital for technicians to take some of Sierra's blood and do a coagulation test.

Having wound our way through the corridors, up the various elevators and into an obscure hallway, we entered the cubicle for blood taking. Sierra's eyes widened as she scanned ominous-looking items of equipment displayed in the room. "What's that for? . . . and that? . . . and that? . . . Are they going to use that on me?"

"I know that one," she said. "That's a butterfly needle for IV."

Sierra sat on my lap, clutched my hand, and watched wisely without a tear as the nurse inserted the dreadful butterfly needle into her vein. *Unbelievable*, I thought as my heart swelled with loving, proud compassion for Sierra. *Those hours of playing with the IV equipment at home have resulted in this composed little girl accepting bravely the thing that had terrified her the most two years ago.*

The technician kept remarking how brave Sierra was, and Sierra said, three or four times, "I'm always brave." Her repeated comments prompted the technician to joke, "Don't break your arm patting yourself on the back."

Equally calmly, Sierra accepted the three sharp pokes on her arm that tested coagulation time. She asked several preparatory questions: "How long will it hurt? How many seconds will it hurt? Tell me again . . . what is it for and what will you do?"

With a warm smile the technician walked us to the elevator and gave Sierra a lollipop. "You ought to wear a sweatshirt, Sierra, that says 'BRAVE KID.'"

"No," said Sierra, "It should say, 'THIS IS A BRAVE KID.'"

In the waiting room at NYU Hospital we met a little girl exactly Sierra's size. We made friendly overtures because we were eager for Sierra to have friends on the ward. When Sierra and Megan each pulled up their shirts to show their Wonder Woman undershirts we chuckled, knowing the connection was made. Through the next three days, Megan and Sierra shared everything.

We were being admitted on March 4th, but Sierra's operation was not scheduled until the sixth. Dr. Doyle had thought the extra day of adjustment would be helpful. Little did we know what was about to happen.

Everything went smoothly through admissions and all procedures on the ward, following roughly the same routine as our admission for catheterization. One new development was that Sierra was beginning to show signs of independence. When the nurse, Rosemary, asked to take

Sierra to be weighed, Sierra took her hand and headed for the door. Some instinct told John and me, without words, not to follow. We both sat still on the windowsill. Realizing we weren't with her, Sierra looked back in a moment of fear, her face asking, "Aren't you coming?" When she saw us calmly beaming at her, we could see the decision being made. Her face changed from fear to surprise and then to pride. She waved goodbye to us. "See you later," she said and stepped out. As they turned the corner, we heard Rosemary say, "You know, I like you."

Rosemary gave her a bath and then took her to see the intensive care unit where Sierra would be the day after her operation. Sierra had little to say about it, although, or perhaps because, she had seen some very sick people and lots of strange beeping machines.

During the evening we all just played together and made more friends on the ward.

The next morning Sierra watched her neighbor receive two shots that made her scream, and then saw her unable to go to sleep before they wheeled her off to the operating room. Then she went to watch Megan get her shots and be wheeled off for her operation.

We played with the other children and received visitors who brought gifts and candy for Sierra and birthday presents for John's birthday. Judy Gueron brought a bag of candy, which made her dear to Sierra's heart forever. Immediately it was shared with all the children on the ward, and still there was enough left for Sierra to have double her quota.

She saved some for Megan, to give her when she returned from the operating room.

Stella sent a roast beef. A whole roast beef, with pumpernickel bread and mustard and a big knife.

Early that evening Sierra started making phone calls to her friends. First Annie. Her side of the conversation went like this:

> Hi . . . fine . . . I'm in the hospital right now but I just wanted to call you up and tell you what's been happening and stuff like that . . . Yes, I had a blood test . . . There were a lot of needles, four needles . . . The nurse did a lot of pokes—very fast—three pokes, one second on each of them since there were three needles . . . And you know those IV needles? They put one into my vein then they took a lot of blood—four tubes of it.

She was interrupted then for her temperature and pulse; when she returned to the phone, Annie had been replaced by her mother. Sierra carried on:

> Well, I haven't finished yet . . . Let Annie tell it to you after . . . OK, see, they did one poke with the butterfly IV needle and then what they did . . . No . . . I'm having a heart operation but it's not in the heart. Sasha had open heart surgery. I'm not having open heart in my heart. What I'm having is . . . I have a narrowing of my aorta. My aorta . . . I don't know . . . It's some part of your body but I don't know where it is . . . What? . . . I know, but . . . Well, that's it I gotta tell you . . . That's it . . . That's about it . . . goodbye.

Then she called Lisa immediately after and started over:

> Hi . . . Fine . . .OK . . . I'm at the hospital right now . . . No, tomorrow they're going to do it . . . Well, have you any questions? . . . Well you might after I tell you this part. See they did a blood test. They drew blood . . . Well, see they had to get some blood from my body because they're going to study it and see if there's any germs in it . . . Have you any questions now . . . You are? . . . The first day I get out? . . . Ask your parents right now . . . Have you anything to tell me? I don't have anything to tell you . . . Well, you know what? I might bring some toys to your house, if I ever go to your house again.

If I ever go to your house again . . .

If I ever go to your house again. That one rung in my ears. Then she called Naveed and started again, in a shortened version:

"Hi . . . have you any questions? No . . . See I'm going to have my operation . . . Well, you know what? Did you know that yesterday I had a blood test? . . . What? . . . I know what a blood test is too, you know why . . ." (She turned to me and asked me what it was really called.) "It's really a coagulation test." Then she went through an elaborate and secret kissing ritual in which they sent each other kisses over the phone.

By about nine p.m. Sierra began to get fussy. She refused to take the little bandage off her blood test without a tape remover. Every little thing became an issue. I decided to help her get at her feelings, so in a high-pitched smiling voice I said, "No! No! No!" Immediately afterward she said "No! No! No!" just as I had, and then she commented, "I think there's something going on with me. I keep wanting to say no."

Continuing, I said it again. She started banging on the curtain around the bed, saying, "No! Don't hurt me! Nothing! Nothing!" She went on for about a minute then asked me to carry her to the bathroom to "Do pee pee." I picked her up and she said, "*Ga ga.*" I naturally responded to her need to be completely taken care of as if she was a baby by saying, "Good baby. Good baby." This delighted her, as it always delights a small child whose parents notice that she needs to be given some special baby attention.

In the bathroom her conversation jumped all over the place. "I just don't want to look in the mirror."

"Why?" I asked

"Because I might look strange."

"You look fine."

"I mean after the operation I might look strange . . ."

I tried to reassure her. "But Sierra those other people are having an operation because they look strange. They don't look strange because they had the operation."

"Oh yeah," she said. "I got it all mixed up. I am all mixed up."

"You've seen a lot of things today," I said.

"I looked at that little boy. I got used to him. I just kept looking."

We kept talking and then John took Sierra for a ride in a wheelchair. There was no possibility of getting her to fall asleep. One of us asked if there were anything else she needed to know before the next day.

"I don't know. Any new surprises. Anything I don't know."

"Well, shall we go over the whole thing with you?"

"Just what I don't know."

"I guess I don't know which things you know and which things you've forgotten. Anyway, I have quite a bit more information than I did two days ago."

"Tell me it."

"OK," I said, "Let's go over it all."

Perhaps I needed to go over it all more than she did. Nonetheless, once we began it seemed the right thing to do, and Sierra's tension seemed to drain away as she heard the reality of what she would face. Many fears and fantasies had been stimulated during this day on the ward.

"Tomorrow morning," I began, "they'll give you the two shots, but you won't have any food, even if you wake up thirsty or hungry. The two shots will be different medications, so we don't know if it'll be two big syringes, one big and one little or two little. But it'll feel the same."

"Oh."

"So, after you go to sleep, they'll put you on the rolling bed."

"I'll be on a rolling bed the whole time or on an operating table."

"Right. They'll take you downstairs after we wave goodbye."

"And," John added, "They'll take you to Dr. Cantor."

"Dr. Cantor?" Sierra asked.

"The anesthesiologist," John said. "He'll give you the mask."

"If I'm not asleep he'll make me blow up a balloon."

"Who told you that?"

"Megan."

"Well, if you're asleep or not, he'll explain everything to you," said John. "So even though you won't be aware of it, someone will still be explaining."

"The mask," Sierra continued offering her new information, "will feel funny. It'll smell funny."

Always eager to give her the full warning, I added, "And it might feel weird because it'll put you to sleep in a different way, kind of quickly. Rebecca said it was yukky."

"She did? Maybe it was because of the smell."

"Maybe so. Then when you're unconscious they'll put you on the operating table," John went on.

"Do it," said Sierra.

Once again, we played out the whole operation, with John being reassuring and making lots of jokes, and me warning of the difficulties, while Sierra alternated between listening intently and laughing uproariously.

John turned her on her side and said, "OK, now get ready to cut, right here."

I jumped up, "Remember, I'm the nurse who takes the pictures." I took some pictures then, but unfortunately none of them came out. John played out the cutting part over and over and then Sierra said, "Come on, Mommy, you have to help. You're the nurse." So I joined the game.

"OK," said John. "Here it is. Now I'll just cut this part of the aorta out, up here by the subclavian artery . . ."

"Oh Doctor," I said, "look at that nice big collateral blood vessel."

"Oh yes," he answered. "I'll just sew that up so it doesn't bleed. She has so many beautiful new arteries carrying her blood, she won't need this one."

"There," I said, "that looks good. Now let's sew it up."

"No," said Sierra, tuned in as always. "You forgot to fix the aorta."

"Yes," said John. "Now I'll sew up the aorta, starting on the back and then coming around to the front. OK, there." All the time of course he was working on Sierra under her left arm where the incision would be, and she was giggling.

"Stop giggling, young lady, hold still! Not so much wiggling—this is a delicate operation," said John. Sierra giggled harder and said, "The doctors don't want to make a mess."

"There," said John. "Now that looks fine. It's done. OK, I'll just open these things up so they fit together, put this patch of Dacron on, and we'll be finished."

"Check her vital signs. How's her blood pressure, her pulse . . ."

"Fine."

Somehow the idea of using my sewing machine had come into it, so Sierra had us pretend to sew her up with the sewing machine several times while she laughed and laughed. We were eager for this laughter. It was a release of tension that was very healthy for all of us.

"OK, now, nurse," said John. "We'll stitch up the pleura. Nurse, turn the sewing machine on . . . turn it off!" Sierra laughed some more.

"OK, let's put the tube in here," John said. "Does it go in here . . . or up this way . . . I don't know . . ." He had forgotten to play doctor and was expressing his own uncertainty.

"Just do it," Sierra put in. "Either way."

"OK, the tube is in that will let the blood and other fluids out of the chest."

"What else does she need . . . oh, yes, she has these three IVs . . . now put in the Foley catheter here, so she can pee-pee, now this nose tube, to keep her well drained, push it all the way down. Well, that looks fine. I think it's all done. She'll heal up . . . she'll hurt for a while, but she'll be fine."

By this time Sierra was falling peacefully asleep. Apparently relaxed.

"Oh," said John in a quiet a voice, seeing her drifting off. "We have to put the dressing on . . . all around here. OK, take her to the recovery room. Soon after she wakes up, she'll see her Mommy and Daddy."

She was sound asleep. It was eleven p.m.

This final review of the operation had been very intimate, very much fun, and very much the three of us together. John and I looked at Sierra, and each other, planning to have another baby as soon as Sierra was safely through the crisis.

One of us finally dozed off and the other crept off to the wonderful parents' room down the hall provided by the hospital. Both of us lived in the hospital now.

We felt that everything was perfectly in place. Everything was ready. We were ready, Sierra was ready, the surgeon and the hospital were ready. All signals were beaming green, for go.

We were totally unprepared for the events of the next day.

CHAPTER THIRTEEN

The Collapse

We all woke up on schedule at 7:30 a.m. It was a sunny day. We gathered in Sierra's bedroom, all ready. Sierra's mood was cheerful and calm.

A nurse entered the room with a look of apology flickering on her face. "I'm sorry," she said. "I just got word that Sierra's operation will have to be postponed slightly. Dr. Isom has been called in to the operating room with an infant. It couldn't be helped. Sierra's operation will have to wait until the emergency is over. I don't know exactly when that will be, but just as soon as they are finished with the infant, they will call upstairs and we will let you know. It could be at about eleven. As soon as we know we will come and give Sierra her three shots."

"I don't want three shots." Sierra reacted strongly. "No, I'm supposed to have only two shots. Three shots is too many. Everybody told me two shots."

Three shots! Three shots plus a delay. Here's trouble, we thought. Now what? Nothing to do but try to take it in stride, ride it through, chalk it up to the surprise factor.

"Well," said the nurse, "it's up to the anesthesiologist and he determined there would be three more shots. The third one is an antibiotic to prevent infection. It's essential. There's nothing that can be done about it."

One of us went quickly to research these three shots, but a call to Dr. Doyle and Dr. Cantor yielded no relief. There would be three shots.

Sierra was not happy about the three shots, but she didn't linger on the subject. She followed our lead in trying to wait cheerfully. Soon our friend Tom Roderick arrived. He had expected to be with John and me during our vigil while the operation was performed. Instead he joined us in a long morning of waiting. With an extraordinary outpouring of loving and playful attention, we succeeded in maintaining a high tone all morning: board games, rides in the wheelchair, balloon games, songs, visits to other children, laughter, love, and closeness. The morning ticked on.

It was eleven o'clock. Eleven thirty. Twelve noon. Still Sierra had been allowed nothing to eat or drink. Still she was cheerful. She had slept only eight hours instead of the optimal eleven hours. Still she was joyously entertaining two younger children with a great balloon game on the ward adjacent to ours. We were bouncing balloons all over the place. We had left word that we could be found on this ward. John was playing his guitar and singing to the great delight of the ward staff.

Twelve thirty p.m. One o'clock. The day dragged on. My heart was slowly sinking. This was too long. This was a lot to ask. When would they come?

Abruptly the door to the ward flew open and two nurses fairly leaped through them. "Sierra Stoneman-Bell! Sierra Stoneman-Bell! Where is she? It's time for her to prepare for her operation." There was a frantic tone to their entrance.

We nearly jumped out of our skins. Yikes! What's the rush all of a sudden? We've been waiting six-and-a-half hours.

"Where were you? We've been looking for you," they repeated.

"We've been right here. We left word on the ward. We've been waiting six hours."

"Well come on. The nurse is ready to give Sierra her shots."

"Nooooooo!" A deep wail rose up from Sierra and the dam broke. All her resolve to be brave, all her painstakingly gathered information, all her calm good humor dissolved in an explosion of terror.

"No! No! No! No! No! Not three shots. Not three shots. Not three shots. No! No! No! Not three shots. Not three shots. No! No! No! Not three shots. I won't do it. They can't do it. No! No! No! No! No! Mommmmmmeeeee Noooooooo! Please don't make me do it. No I can't do it. I'm only supposed to have two shots. Not three shots. Pleeeeeeeease, don't make me do it." She sputtered through heavy sobs.

For the next forty minutes we tried to work through Sierra's sudden terror so she could get back on track and accept the shots. Our method would have been to let her panic. Let her cry all the way through and have it out. It was certainly appropriate for her to be upset. Three shots. No food or drink. Little sleep. Tension building for two days. A six-hour wait. Then a mad rush toward the thing she feared the most: shots.

She was entitled to cry and be held and tell us how scared she was and how mad she was about the extra shot. She was four-and-a-half years old.

So we held her, and we listened. We reassured her and encouraged her to take the shots. But this wasn't enough. The heat was really on. The nurses wanted those injections done. They were hovering, moving in, backing off when Sierra redoubled her outcries, cajoling, warning, urging us to hold her arms and legs and do it by force. Time was running out. The rush was on.

We later pieced together what must have happened. The order had gone up from the operating room at 12:45 p.m., but didn't get to us until 1:30 p.m. There had been a precious forty-five minutes lost somewhere, and now it was Sierra who was to make them up.

The nurses were trying to be nice, but it was their job to have the patients prepared for the operating room on schedule. The surgeons are the top of the medical hierarchy. The operating room was in great demand. It is not OK to keep the surgeons waiting and the operating room empty because a patient isn't ready.

A second call was received on the ward: the surgeons were waiting. Where was the patient?

John and I were incapable of changing our mode of dealing with Sierra. We simply could not, and neither could she, switch to a coercive mode at the last minute when the heat was on. Up until now Sierra had been a full partner in everything. She had accepted every procedure willingly, and in this hospitalization she had already accepted an IV needle without a tear or a whimper.

But now she was using her full persuasive force, through piteous pleas and physical resistance, to avoid the third shot. After half an hour of letting her cry and agreeing that it was a terrible surprise and we understood her feelings, she accepted two of the shots. After the second one, which was very painful, her resistance stiffened. More tears, more pleas, “I’m scared, Mommy. It isn’t fair. I’m scared. I don’t want three shots. I don’t even want an operation.”

Ten more minutes ticked past. A small crowd of nurses and residents was gathering. Two surgeons in training arrived from the operating room to see what was holding up the show. On the forty-fifth minute Sierra agreed to the third shot.

I held her and she wept. Then I was called on the phone by Dr. Doyle, calling from the operating room. “Mrs. Stoneman, what’s going on up there.”

“Sierra has just accepted the third shot. It will take a while for the shots to take effect. We don’t want her to go downstairs until she has fallen asleep.”

"All right. Of course, she won't have to go until she's asleep." Relieved, I turned to Sierra and joined John in holding and trying to calm her so the shots would take effect.

It had been an excruciating forty-five minutes.

Sierra said, "I don't want to go downstairs yet. I don't want to go until I'm asleep."

"No, Sierra. You don't have to. We'll stay right here until you are asleep." Dr. Doyle had said so.

Within minutes a masked orderly wheeled the rolling bed directly into Sierra's room and announced, "I must have the patient. She is due in the operating room right now."

"No," we said. "She's not going until she's asleep."

"She must come now."

"She's not asleep. Dr. Doyle told us she didn't have to come until she was asleep. We promised Sierra. She's not going now."

Sierra was screaming and clutching me. "Mommy don't make me go."

The orderly left. Little by little Sierra's little body began to relax in my arms.

Five minutes later he was back, with two surgeons-in-training.

"There are more than a dozen people waiting for you in the operating room. We can't keep the operating room empty any longer. She must come now or there will be no operation."

John and I looked at each other. Sierra jerked awake and grabbed me again, "No, Mommy! I'm not asleep." Her convulsive sobbing started again.

"Well, then," I said. "There will be no operation today." They turned on their heels and strode out.

John and I managed to exchange a few words. We were in agreement. There was no way we would let an orderly or a surgeon yank Sierra out of our arms and drag her kicking and screaming to an operating room and force her to take the anesthesia. This was out of the question.

The nurse summoned me to the phone. It was Dr. Doyle. "Mrs. Stoneman, what is this about not doing the operation today?"

"Dr. Doyle, Sierra is extremely upset. She didn't expect three shots. The medication hasn't taken effect and we promised her she would not go to the operating room until she was asleep. She can't be dragged to the operating room kicking and screaming. It will probably take about a half hour for her to go to sleep and they said they couldn't wait."

"All right. We'll call it off for today. It's not good when a child is hypertense. It's medically contraindicated. You'll have to reschedule it at a time convenient for the surgeon. I'll talk to you later."

She sounded angry, but fundamentally calm and clear.

I rushed back to John and Sierra. "It's off for today. We're not having the operation. We'll have to reschedule it."

"Oh no," said Sierra. "Do we have to do it all over again?"

"Yes."

"Can we wait until I'm five?"

Twenty minutes later Sierra was completely medicated. John and I were completely devastated.

It was unbelievable. The operation was postponed. Was it all our fault? Had we made terrible errors? How come we couldn't force Sierra to take the shots? Why couldn't we get instant obedience in an emergency? Why did we still have to get a four-and-a-half-year-old's consent? Why did we have to let her cry for forty-five minutes? What was wrong with us?

We turned to Tom. He had witnessed the whole thing. What did he think? Had we done the right thing or were we crazy?

Tom is a good friend, and a smart one. No matter what, he would have said we had done the right thing. There is nothing else to say to distraught parents when they have just taken a risky position on a principle that is consistent with all their other child rearing and puts them into a confrontation with the medical establishment. You have to say they did the right thing.

All our friends told us we did the right thing. Every single one of them. We knew they would. Many of them said we were brave, and wonderful, and models for other parents, and that Sierra would never forget how her parents stood up for her in that crisis. Lots of them said it would have been a disaster if we had yielded and betrayed Sierra after so much careful preparation.

They all said it wasn't our fault.

But we felt terrible. After all, it was an absolute privilege to have access to the best medical care in the world. What right did we have to violate that privilege because of something so trivial and predictable as feelings of fear in a child?

We knew what our friends would say. We were grateful to them. But the biggest reassurance of all came from an unexpected source. That evening the head nurse who hadn't been on the ward in the afternoon stopped John in the hallway. "What happened?" she asked sympathetically. He explained.

"You did the right thing," she said. John burst out crying in relief and gratitude, and the nurse kindly hugged him.

CHAPTER FOURTEEN

The Aftermath

AFTER WRITING NUMEROUS DRAFTS, trying to make each one simpler, shorter, and less laden with feeling than the previous one, I managed to come up with a one-page letter to the doctors that I hoped expressed a balanced perspective on what had happened. On March 8th, I sent off the following letter:

Dear Dr. Kantor and Dr. Isom:

We're sorry and sad about the costly and inconvenient postponement of Sierra's surgery, but we know that worse things happen every day and that it wasn't anyone's fault. The main factors causing it seemed to be:

-the rescheduling from morning to afternoon of the surgery;

-the addition of a third injection to the two that Sierra expected;

-an apparent delay in the order reaching us (we understand that the order went up from the operating room at about 12:15, but it was after 1:00 p.m. when it reached us);

-a sudden caving in of Sierra's previously apparent resolve to be brave when an upsurge of fear overtook her;

-an inability on our part to shift from a consensual approach with Sierra to a coercive one, even though time constraints were indicating it might be necessary;

-time pressures on the surgical team and the operating room, making it impossible to wait for Sierra to calm down and go to sleep (She was finally asleep, fully medicated, at 3:30 p.m.. It would have been sooner without the many interruptions after she had accepted the three shots).

We appreciated that nobody insulted us or tried to force us during the incident. It was very difficult as it was, but any of the medical staff could have made it a lot worse, and none did.

We look forward to our all trying again, successfully, and as Dr. Doyle put it, "playing our cards differently." We consider it a privilege to have access to the excellent medical care you are providing. We want you to know that we don't take it lightly, in case you were wondering what in the world we thought we were doing up there while you all were waiting downstairs.

We agree with Dr. Doyle's suggestion about next time: that it be first thing in the morning, with only two shots given at the same time, with the morphine given first and the antibiotic given in the operating room. We would add that if it is possible to diminish the shots even to one, or to an oral sedative, that would be good, but in any case we think there should be plenty of time for the sedative to take effect before Sierra is taken downstairs.

We are eager to get it over with, as you can imagine.

Sincerely yours,
John Bell, Dorothy Stoneman

cc: Dr. Eugenie Doyle

****

It was our wish to get it over with; but it was Sierra's heartfelt wish to wait until she was five. The doctors granted Sierra her desire, unwittingly, by rescheduling the operation for May 26th. Eleven weeks away.

Eleven weeks loomed ahead like an eternity. There was nothing for us to do but go back to our regular lives. Back to work. Back to school. Forget about the whole thing.

We tried to do just that, with reasonable success. I kept no notes of those eleven weeks, and whatever happened during them regarding the operation, or Sierra's anticipation of it, is forever lost in our memories, except for one general change in our parenting.

There was just one element of preparation we systematically did in those eleven weeks. Having decided that whatever happened, we needed to be in a position to "call the shots" (in a manner of speaking), getting obedience from Sierra if her life depended on it even if she didn't like the idea, we had been much stricter parents for eleven weeks. If we asked her to do something, we required obedience rather than negotiation. Any resistance on her part was met by our counting to ten, slowly out loud, and then forcing her to do what we asked. Usually the issue was minor, like putting on a coat or cleaning something up or taking a bath. But the weight behind our parental feeling that we had to be able to get instant obedience next time was enormous. Sierra hated this new and seemingly unnecessary struggle that we would impose on her at every hint of resistance. But after eleven weeks, she did, indeed, believe that there was no point in negotiating or resisting if we once started counting.

My work reabsorbed me. I faced up to the need to fire a well-loved staff member whose incompetence was threatening our entire project. This was something I had avoided for quite a while, because I hate conflict and I liked the person in question. But my assistant and I knuckled down and did the terrible deed, despite the picketing of our offices by irate young people who loved the staff member and couldn't believe he was at fault for a whole long list of failures in the project. Some irrational and anonymous person even called my office threatening to kill me if I really fired this guy.

After the crisis was over, I woke up on an April weekend to a lovely, warm, sunny day with spring all through the air. Bouncing out of bed, I announced to John that I was going to do something I'd never indulged in before, because it had always been simply too expensive and luxurious. I was going to rent a horse to ride in Central Park, to enjoy the great cascades of cherry tree blossoms and the delicious smell of spring. I planned to canter alone and free along the paths, like a young girl on her dream horse.

At the Eighty-Sixth Street stable the young man led out a very large chestnut gelding. As I leaped up to his back, in a motion unfamiliar for many years, something snapped in my back, and I felt a searing pain in my lower left side. Unwilling to cancel my fantasy ride, I carried on with it, getting stiffer and stiffer at every moment, until the hour was over and I could barely dismount without being lifted from the horse's back.

By nightfall I was immobilized on the floor of our bedroom, curled up in a muscle spasm that prevented me from moving without intense pain. For two weeks I lay on my back, slowly healing, theorizing that the combination of pressure at work and anxiety about the operation had finally brought me down. So I rested, and like so many people before me, determined to do daily back exercises for the rest of my life, in a regimen designed to heed God's warning that I was pushing my limits and should take better care of myself.

Photo Album

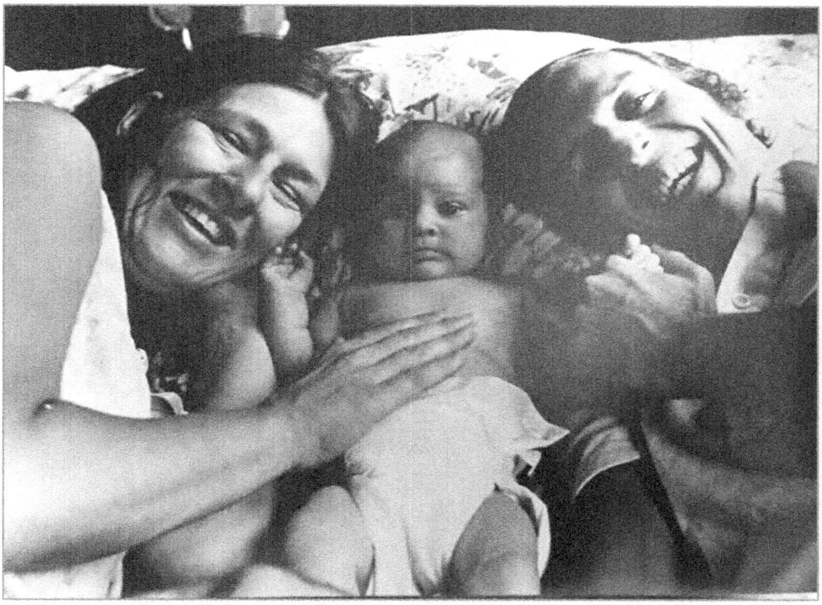

It's 1976. John and I are delighting in our wonderful baby.

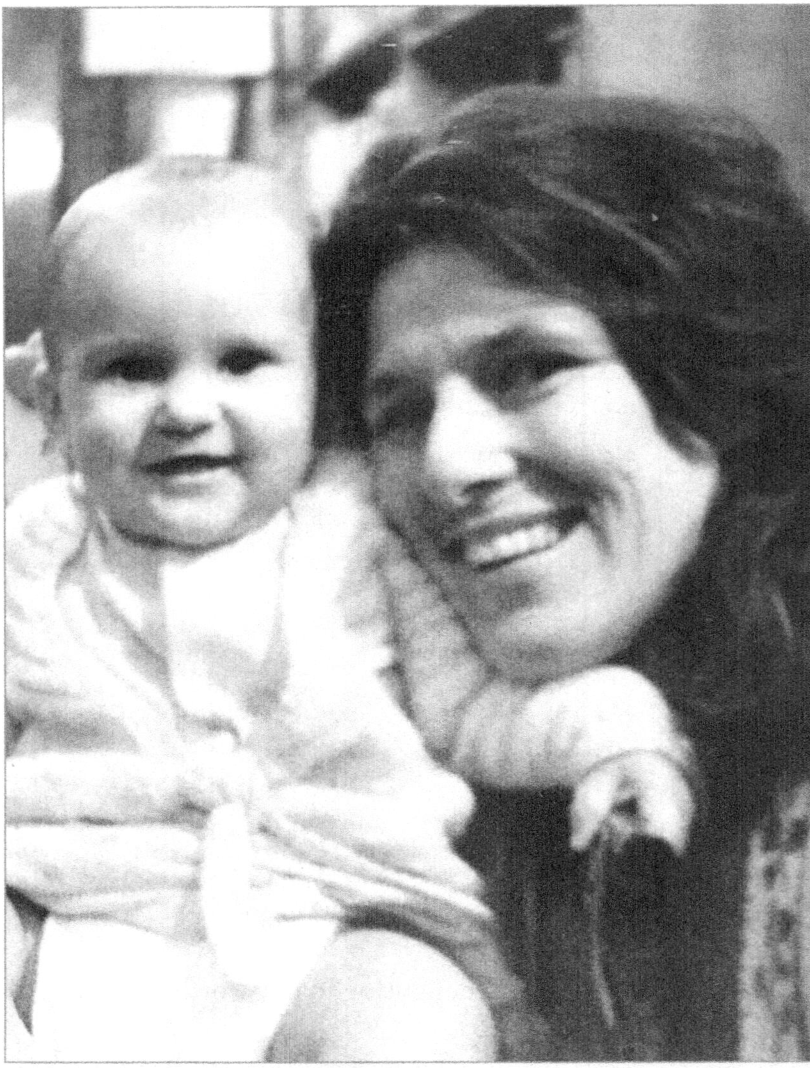

I love being Sierra's mother!

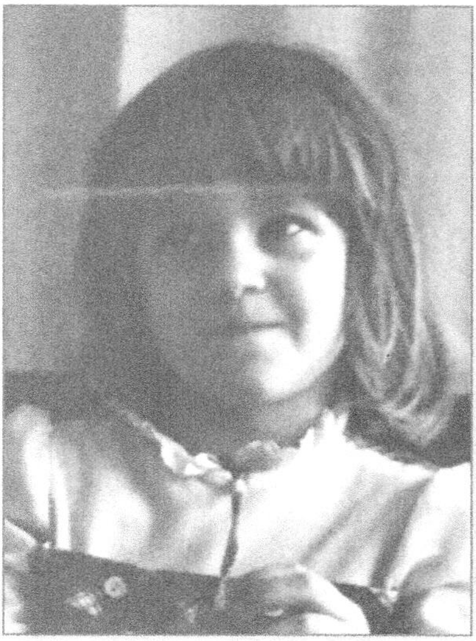

Sierra is about four years old. She is so sweet, so very open to learning and thinking.

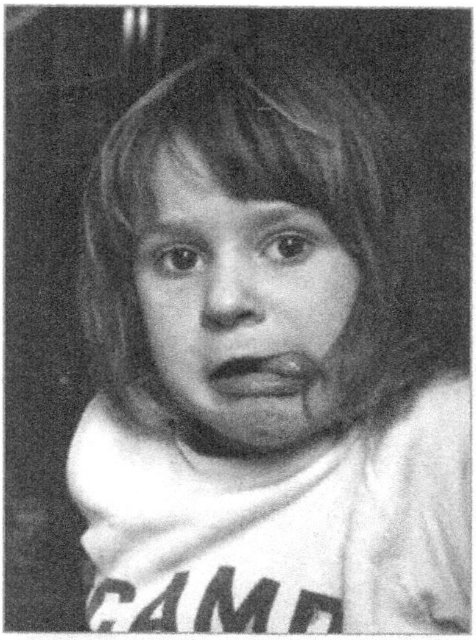

Sierra is not so pleased with whatever she just heard!

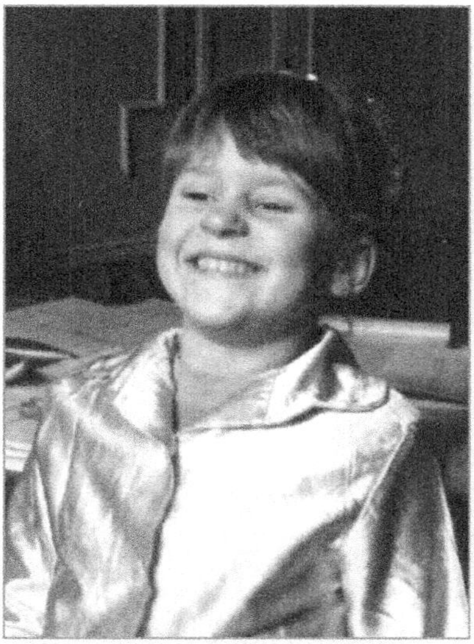

She is working hard to be ready for whatever she has to face.

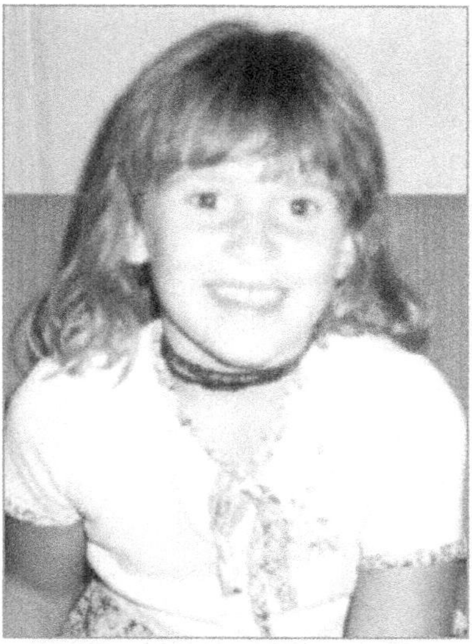

Now Sierra is fully prepared, all ready to go to the hospital!

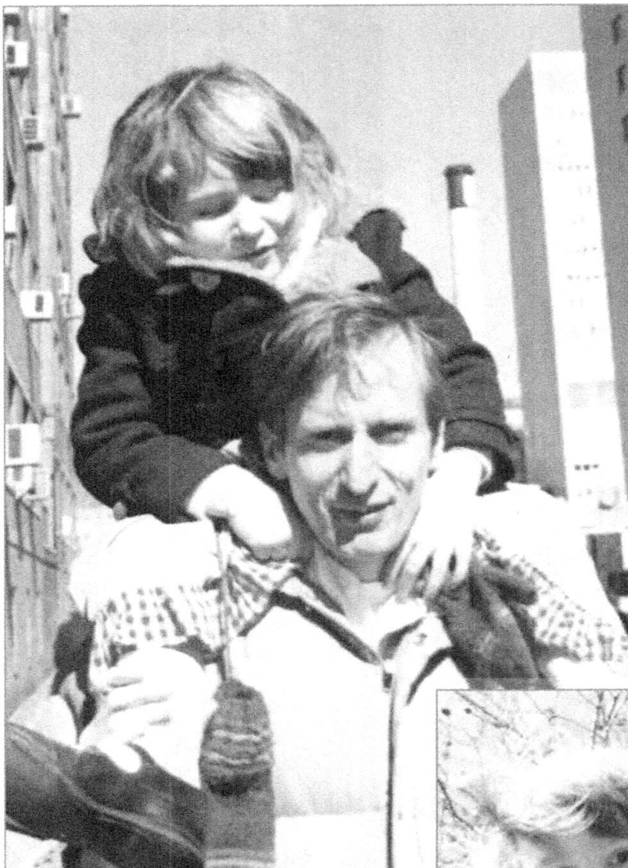

Sierra is riding on John's shoulders as they walk to the hospital.

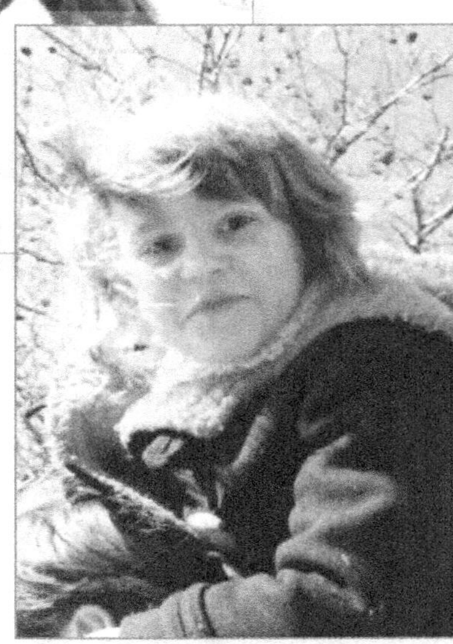

She fully enjoys the walk to the hospital on John's shoulders. The sun is out and she is ready!

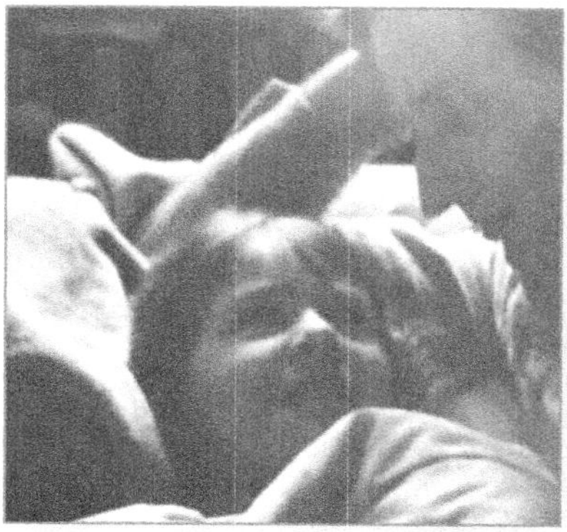

Sierra looks trustingly up at her dad in the hospital bed. They are preparing to dramatize the operation.

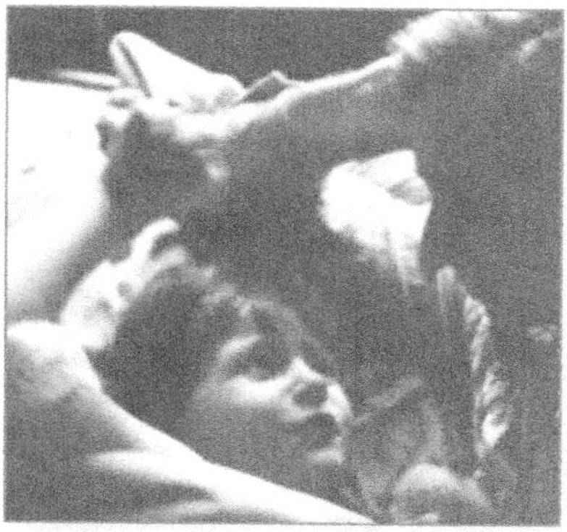

The game begins! John pretends to be the doctor.

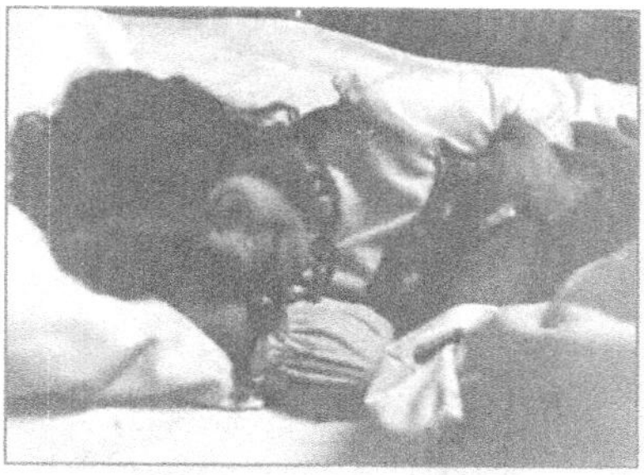

John reaches for her chest while Sierra resists, with a smile on her face.

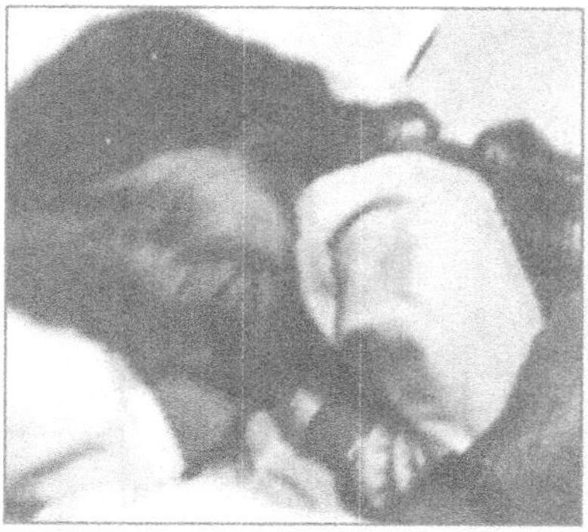

Sierra thinks it's funny and laughs hard!

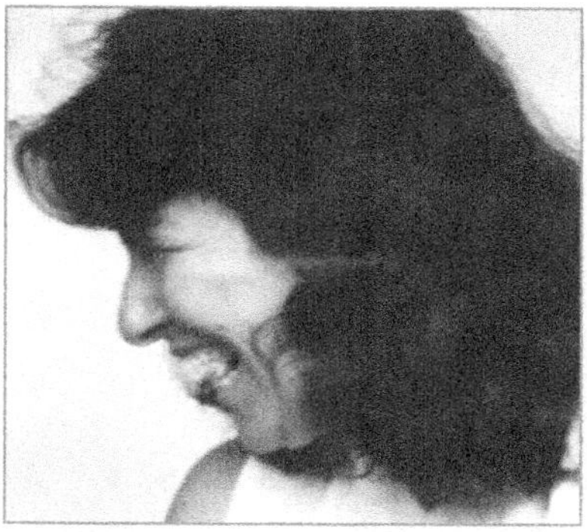

I think it's funny too!

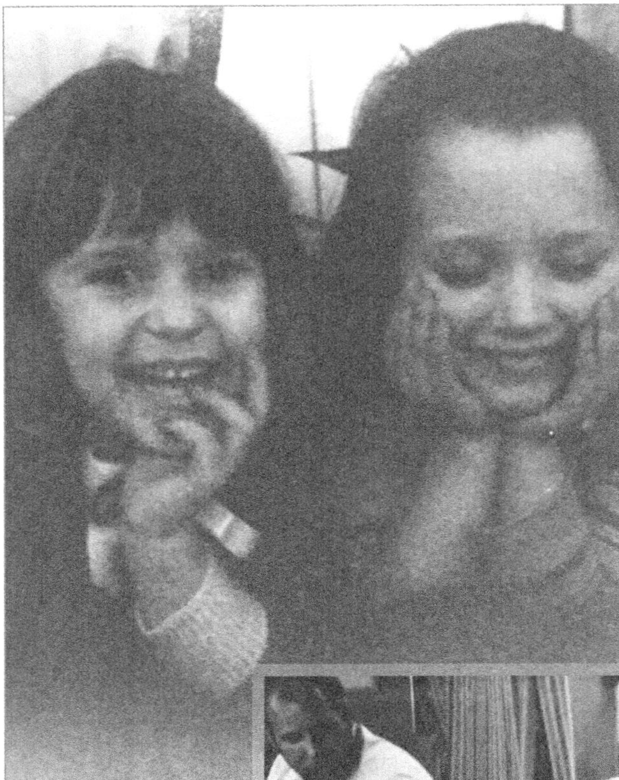

Sierra and her good friend share feelings about doctors and hospitals.

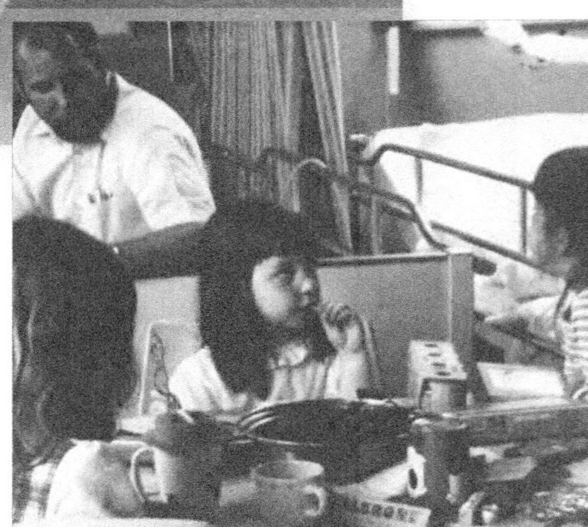

The children in the hospital play together.

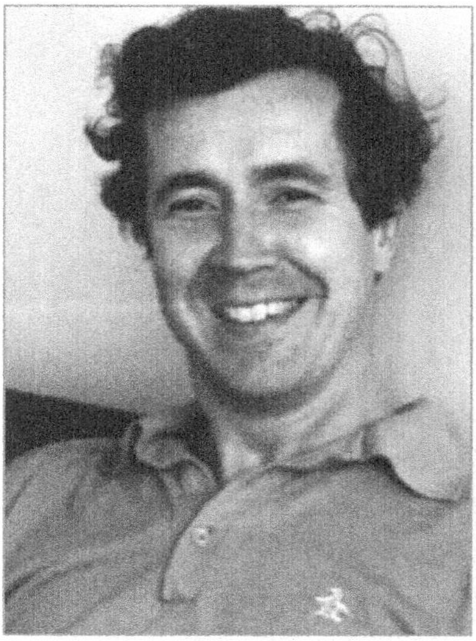

Our friend Tom Roderick sits in the waiting room with us while Sierra undergoes her surgery.

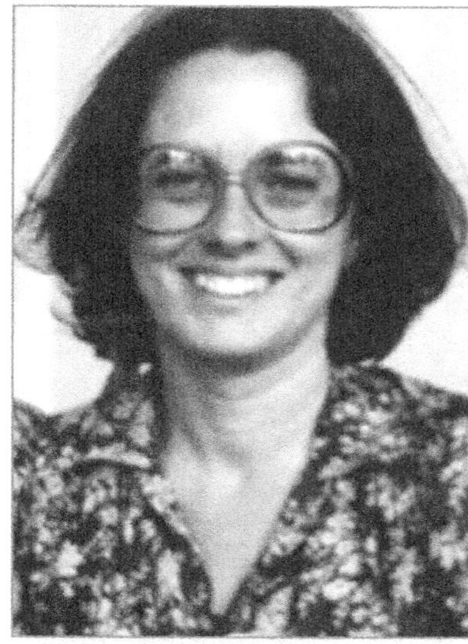

Our friend Lisel Burns is also with us in the waiting room.

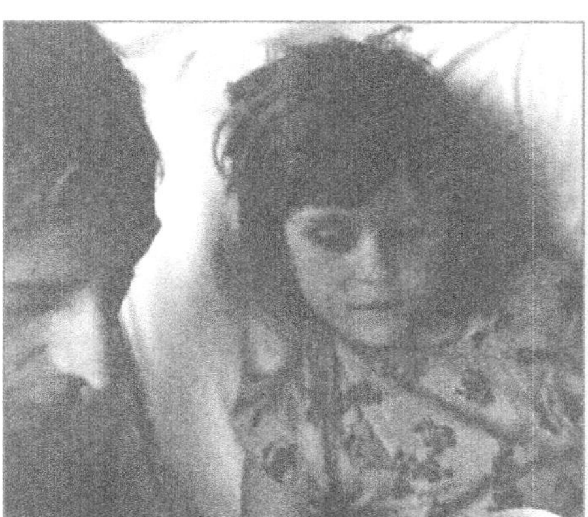

After the surgery, Sierra and John share a book.

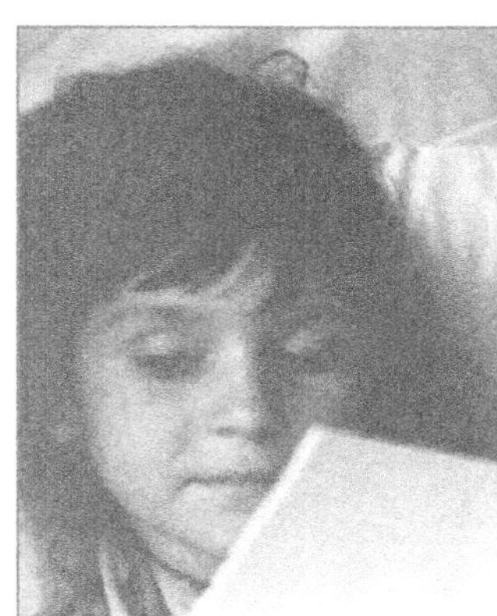

Sierra peacefully enjoys the book.

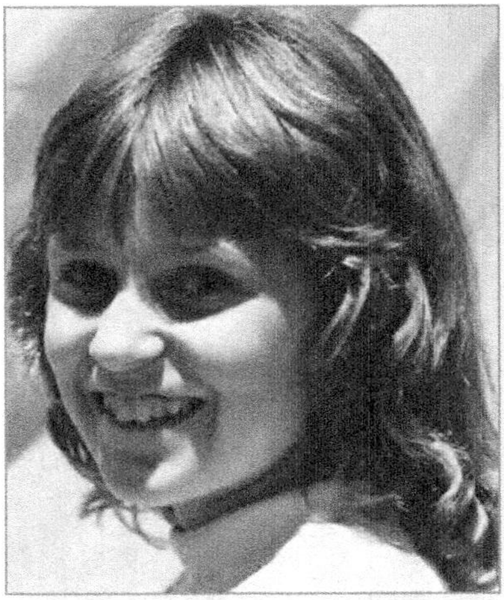

This is Sierra a couple years after surgery, fully recovered.

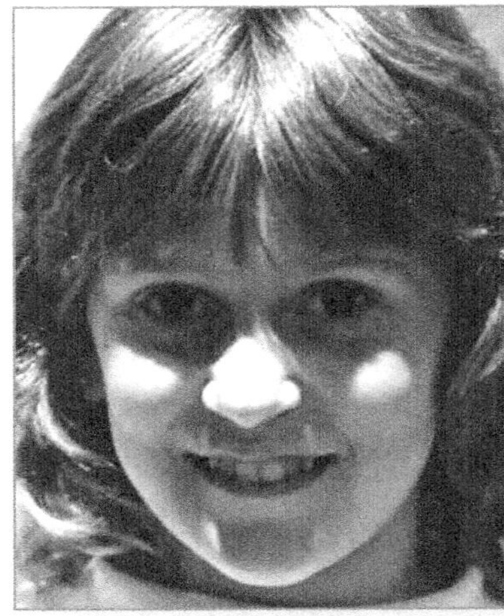

She is ready for the rest of her life!

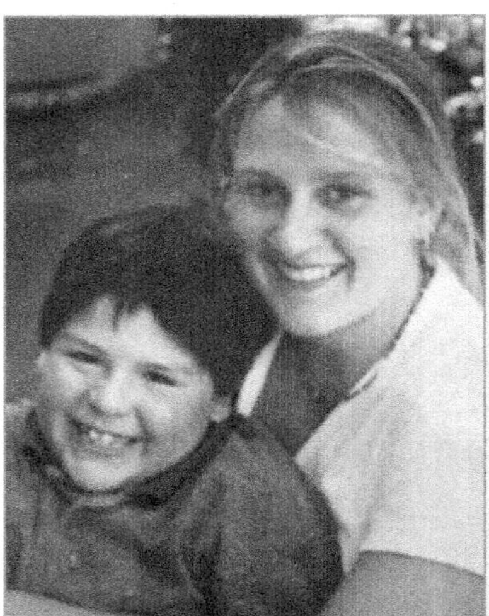

When Sierra is twelve years old, we adopt a wonderful new baby. His name is David Lautaro Stoneman-Bell (nicknamed Taro). Here they are, loving each other, when he was about five and she was about seventeen.

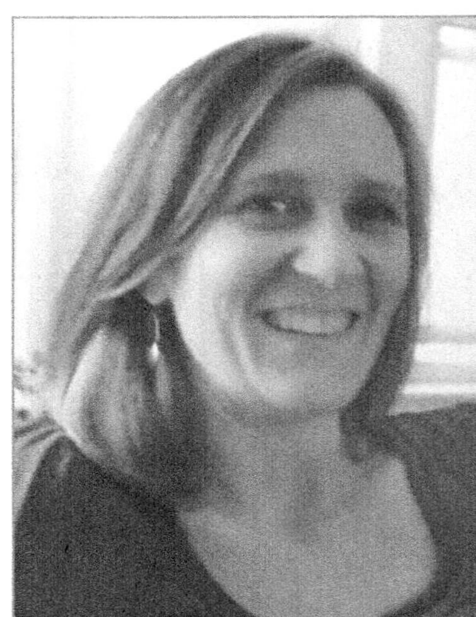

Sierra's heart stays healthy as she grows into a happy and beautiful young adult.

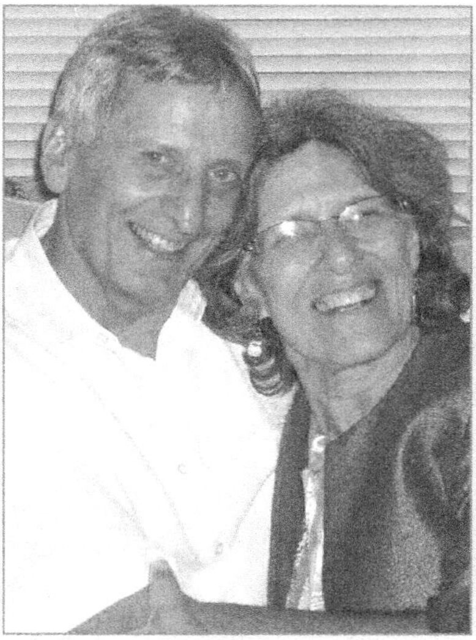

John and I stay happily together.

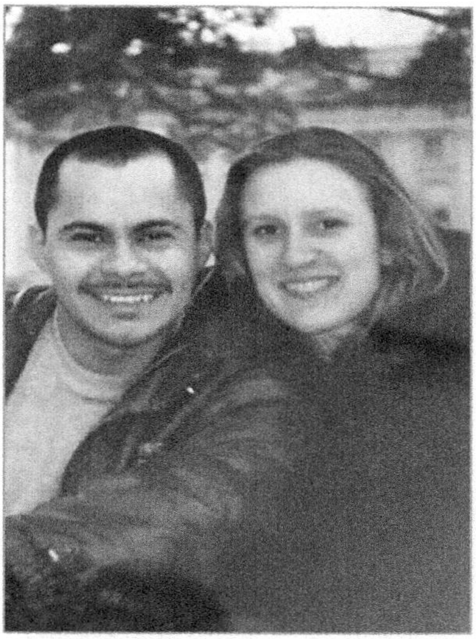

Sierra falls in love with Fernando Aguilera.

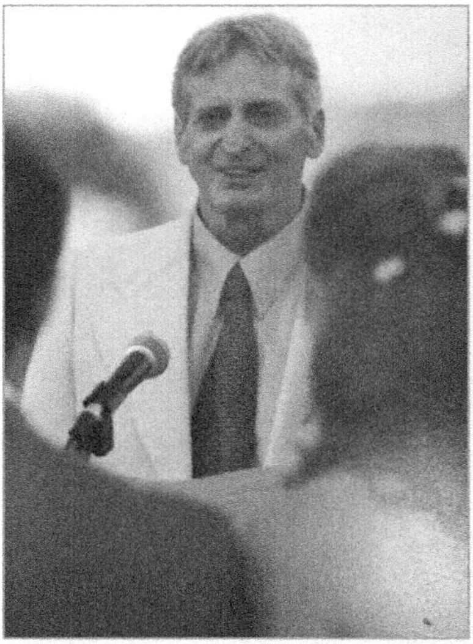

Sierra and Fernando get married. John speaks at their wedding.

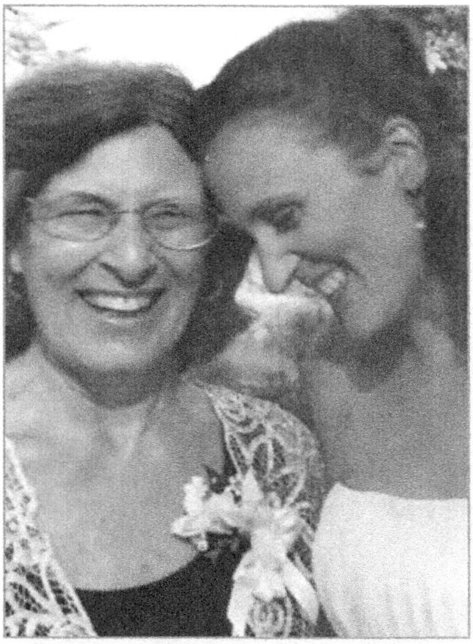

Sierra and I are happy together at her wedding!

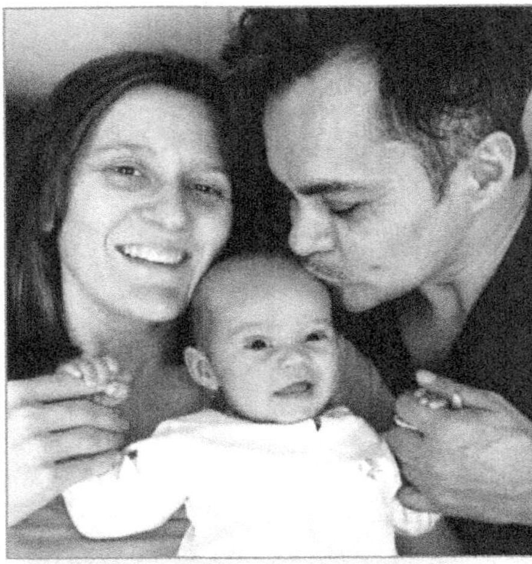

Soon Sierra and Fernando have their own wonderful baby, named Antu. In the language of the Mapuche, the indigenous people of Chile, Fernando's home country, Antu means "great spirit of the sun."

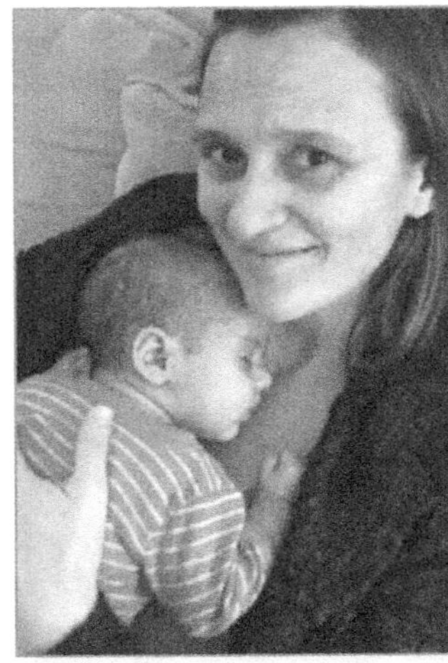

Sierra loves being Antu's mom as much as I loved being her mom!

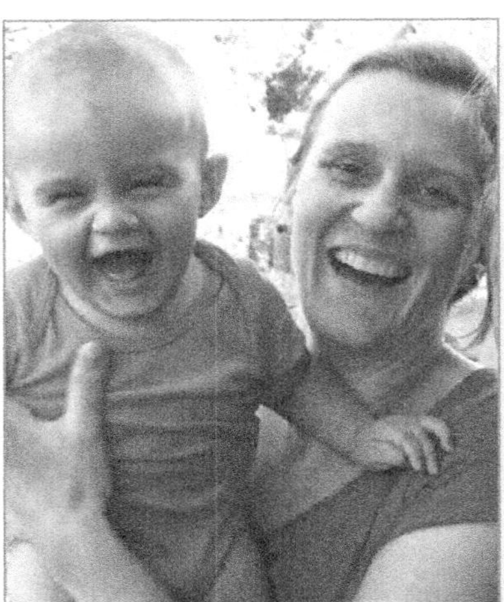

How happy they are!

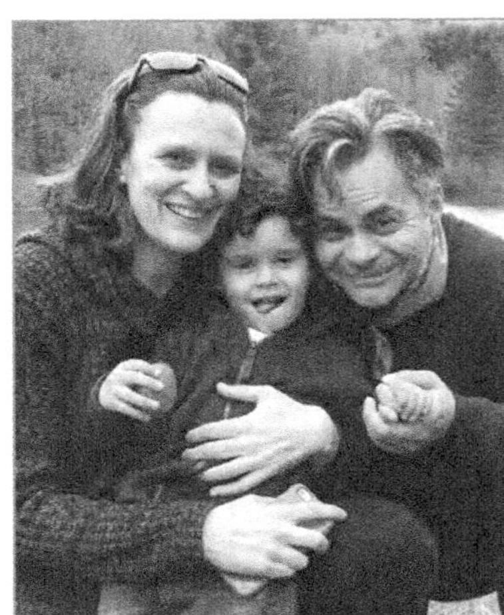

Now Antu is five. He does not have a coarctation of the aorta and will not need surgery!

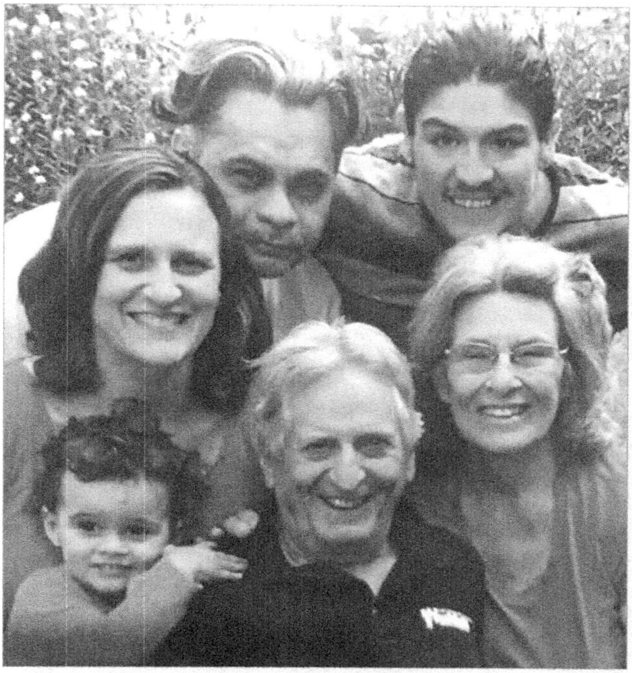

Our family is happy and healthy together:
Sierra, Fernando, Taro, Dorothy, John, and Antu!

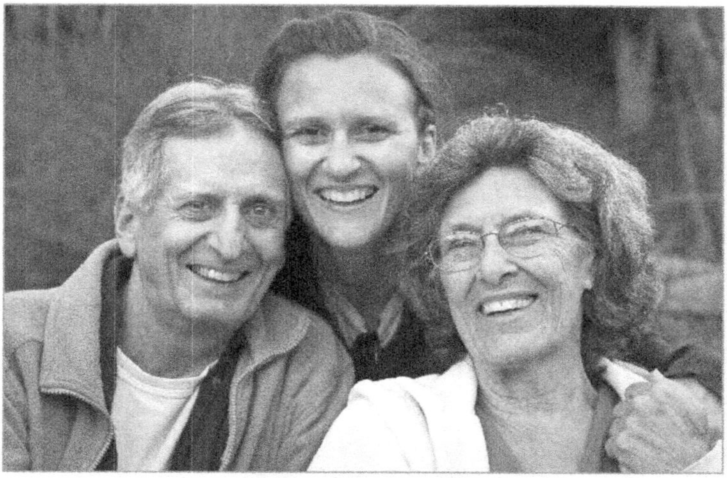

Here we are, happy and grateful,
thirty-five years after the operation.

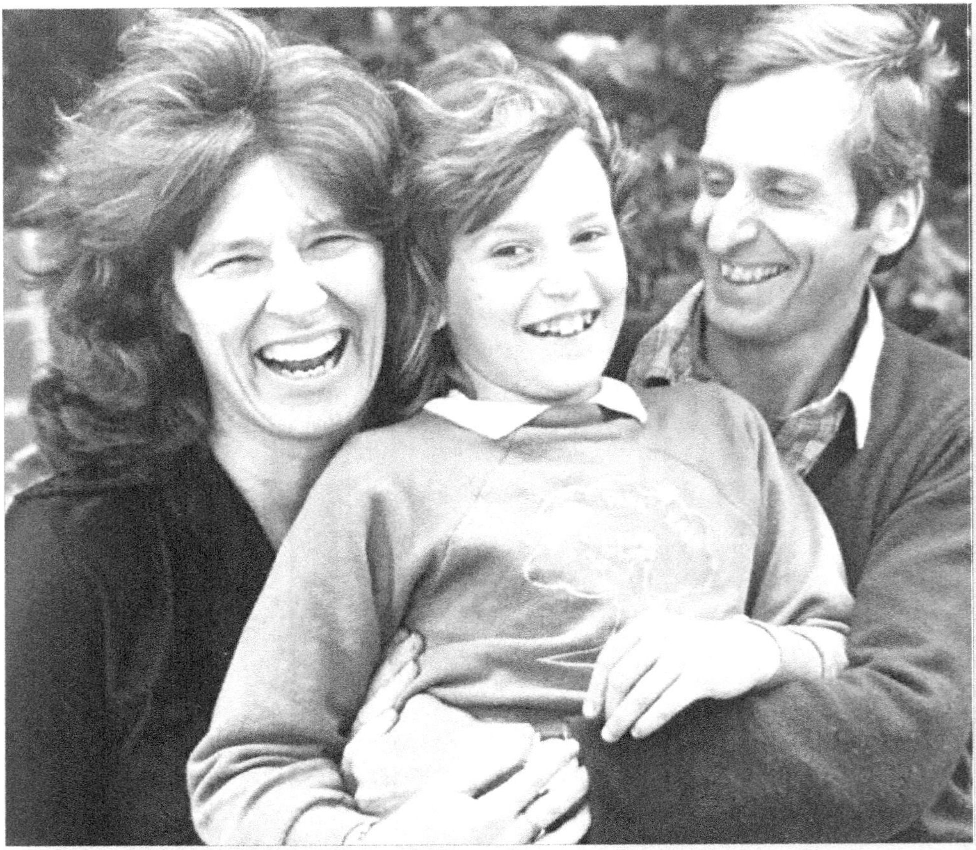

CHAPTER FIFTEEN

Try Again

It was approaching the end of May. The operation surfaced again, taking over our consciousness. This time we thought we would just take it in stride, making no big deal about it. In a demonstration of relaxation, we went car camping for a family outing three days before the scheduled hospitalization.

The next morning Sierra woke up with a tiny cough. At every cough, John and I looked despairingly at each other. Should we have gone camping? Now will she get a cold? Have we been negligent again, doing this stupid thing of going camping so close to hospitalization? We had to keep reminding ourselves that for eleven weeks Sierra had been in perfect health, with no effort whatsoever on our part. We never made her wear warmer clothes than she wanted, and we let her stay up as late as she wanted. There was no reason to think she needed any special protection to stay healthy. Sleeping in a car under a blanket on a warm spring night should not give her a cold.

But she kept coughing, and sniffling. On Tuesday morning we called Dr. Doyle and Rodney and told them both we were not sure if Sierra was coming down with a cold or not, but we were concerned. Rodney saw her on Tuesday, listened to her chest, and pronounced her in fine health. He said he had no way of knowing if she were about to come down with a cold, but at this moment she had no congestion. Seeing John's worried face, Rodney put his arms around John and hugged him, "She's going to be fine."

At dinnertime Sierra continued to sniffle. Tim asked her if she was getting a cold. "I don't know." Then Tim asked, "Do you want to get this cold?" With her deep silence, typical when something was emotion laden, she nodded her head in a slight yes.

Between three a.m. and nine a.m. Sierra coughed fifty-three times. In the morning we started timing her coughs. They were coming once every four minutes, on average, with the longest interval between coughs being fifteen minutes. We tried to hide from her that we were writing it down every time we heard her cough, but she was quite curious about the little piece of paper with the numbers all over it.

John kept saying, "I don't like it. I don't like it. She's not in her best of health. She's not ready for a big operation. She's definitely getting a cold."

I kept saying, "I think it's all right. I think it's all right."

Sierra kept coughing, every four minutes.

John called Dr. Doyle and asked if she would take a look at Sierra prior to admission, just to check if she had any congestion. She said, "It's a bad day, but come to my office at Bellevue at one o'clock, and I'll take a look. You don't have to get a new coagulation blood test, because the one from three months ago will suffice. But come to my office for a little checkup."

As we drove downtown on the East River Drive, we conversed about how long people live. Sierra said, "Heidi's grandmother lived to be one hundred and nine. That's the oldest." John said, "I'm going to live forever." Sierra said, "One thing is for sure. I'm going to live longer than either of you, because I'm younger and I was born later." By the end of the conversation we had mentioned the ages of all the other people we knew. Once again, I wondered if Sierra had any foreboding. I wondered if she had any idea the operation could be life threatening. It was the one thing we had chosen never to share with her.

At Bellevue, I bought her a little chocolate egg, like the one she had wanted so desperately in March. She was delighted when I said, "I'll keep it in my pocketbook and pull it out sometime in the hospital when you really need a surprise."

Sierra had chosen to bring two toys with her to the hospital: her doll, Karen; and her pencil sharpener, which was a tiny little globe of the world. I was surprised, and pleased, that she was taking the whole world along with her. We sat on some stairs inside Bellevue waiting for John to park the car. She pulled out her little globe and asked, "Where is New York?" I showed her, and then she said, "But where is Asia?" At that moment two nurses, one of them Asian, were walking by. She flashed us a broad smile, hearing Sierra's question. I liked it. I always like any contact that links people across the racial barriers that have been placed between different peoples.

In the examining room, Dr. Doyle listened to Sierra's chest, "She has no congestion, but she does have a little sniffle. It's not optimal, but there's no risk. I think we can go ahead."

"If it's not optimal," one of us said, "Wouldn't it be just as easy to wait until next week?"

"Let me call Dr. Isom and check on his schedule."

She strode back a few minutes later saying, "I reached Dr. Isom in Boston. There is a possibility that the Hospital Workers Union will go on strike on Monday. That means if we put it off it may not happen at all next week or the week after. Mrs. Stoneman, you're on leave again from your work?" I nodded. She looked at John and Sierra, then said firmly, "Mr. Bell," knowing he was the most hesitant this time, "I think we should go ahead." With a decisive thrust of her arm she said emphatically, "Let's go!"

"You think we should?"

"Yes, I do."

"Well, then. OK. Let's go."

Dr. Doyle handed us Sierra's medical record, and said, chuckling, "Please give this to the resident on the ward when you get over there. I didn't want to send it over until I was sure Sierra would really be admitted."

So, the die was cast. If Dr. Doyle said it was OK, then it must be OK.

"One more question, Dr. Doyle. If Sierra starts coughing tonight on the ward, what do we do?"

"We reconsider."

"But who do we tell? Do we call you?"

"No, tell the resident on duty. She'll call me."

We said goodbye and slowly wandered to the elevator looking at everything as we went. Dr. Doyle turned out to be also on the elevator so we crowded in next to her. As the elevator descended Sierra began to cough. It was the thickest and most persistent cough she'd had since the night before. My eyes met Dr. Doyle's. She raised her eyebrows significantly.

She turned to Sierra, with some humor and I thought some hope that Sierra's cough was deliberate and therefore no problem. "Sierra, that's some cough." I quickly told Dr. Doyle that Sierra had not been capable of producing a cough on demand the day before when I had asked her to cough for Rodney. When the elevator reached the ground floor, we all disembarked and said goodbye with tentative smiles and hopeful looks.

At New York University Medical Center, we got through admissions in record time, with only one surprise: we were on the west ward, where they had no telephones. I interpreted the lack of telephones as a kind of discrimination against parents and a lack of awareness about the needs of children. Of course, small children in the hospital would like to hear from their friends on the telephone, and of course parents would be eager to use the phone.

I still didn't feel at all nervous. It seemed like I had exhausted and discharged my anxiety the last time. Now it seemed all pretty matter of fact. But John was tense, still worried about the cold.

On the ward we were rooming with a little boy named Peter who was three years old and was recovering from heart surgery done the week before. Dr. Isom and Dr. Doyle were his doctors also. John engaged his mother in conversation about how wonderful the doctors were, while I played with Sierra.

When Sierra and I returned, John was in a deep conversation with an anesthesiologist who would handle our case the next day. Yogi, the doctor, was explaining that there would have to be three shots the next day, as before, because some of the medications couldn't be mixed.

I was shocked. Why couldn't they get their act together? We must have talked to Yogi for half an hour. Then he knelt down and said to Sierra, "Sierra, there will have to be three shots tomorrow. Can you handle that?" She said, simply, "Yes."

Two minutes later the resident on the ward arrived with her tourniquet and needle to take blood for the blood test. Sierra dissolved in sobs, grabbing my legs, saying, "No! No! No! No! . . . wait . . . no, I don't want it . . . No! No! No!" This was all too familiar.

John and I went into our counting routine. Whatever had happened before, this time Sierra must be able to obey despite her fears. It worked; she submitted.

Sure enough, somehow the three shots were still necessary, despite the best of intentions. Nonetheless, we had a restful evening, reviewing with Sierra some of what to expect, and mostly chatting with other people on the ward.

The next morning dawned bright and sunny, with all of us up and ready for the nurse, who came right on schedule, and administered the shots while we firmly counted to ten on each one. Sierra shed no tears. She gripped our fingers, looked squarely at the long needles, and didn't flinch. Within twenty minutes she was asleep, and was rolled away on the bed.

John and I fled to the parents' room, where our friends Tom Roderick and Lisel Burns were prepared to share with us the long wait through the fateful hours of surgery. For hours we talked, and wept, and prayed, and made jokes, and looked nervously at our watches. It was good to be with such close friends to fill the endless time and carry some of the burden of suspense.

Three-and-a-half hours later Dr. Doyle appeared in the parents' room. "The operation is complete. All went well. We did not have to use a patch. She'll be in the recovery room within a half hour. You can relax now."

Jubilation.

CHAPTER SIXTEEN

The Recovery Room

THE NEXT TWENTY-FOUR HOURS were anything but relaxing. This was the long-awaited period of Sierra being in the recovery room. The deal had been that we could be in there with her, but it was not so simple. We had to use all our wiles to get in and stay in. Waiting patiently, sneaking in, being helpful, being invisible, disappearing at critical moments, returning unobtrusively, befriending nurses, hiding from the head nurse, being put out at the changing of the shifts and starting all over again: it was an ordeal. Of the twenty-four hours Sierra spent in the recovery room, we were only able to maneuver our way to her bedside for eight of those hours. The eight hours were not consecutive hours. In and out, dodging the disapproving ones and sidling back in when the approving ones were on duty, it was a constant struggle. Pacing the halls, ranting and raving at. the injustice of it and the frustration, not being able to anticipate when they would let us in and when they wouldn't: it was completely unnecessary torture.

Whenever we did get in, we would make ourselves useful, standing silently by Sierra's bed and calming her. The nurses said Sierra was clearly calmer when we were there, yet it was common hospital lore that parents make the children more upsettable.

In the recovery room Sierra had a nurse at her side at every moment, monitoring her blood pressure, her medication, her drainage tubes. She was awake and alert. When she first woke up, she gazed around and said, "No more shots." Then, when there was a shot she had to have in the recovery room she said, "Let me give it to myself. Let my Mommy or Daddy do it."

This continued for the next few days. She didn't want anybody doing anything to her. "Don't touch me." "Not so fast." "Let my Mommy or Daddy do it." "I'll do it myself." and "No." These were her comments. She had had it with doctors and nurses doing these things to her.

This was the only symptom she had of what the hospital termed "post-cardiac personality." According to hospital workers, after cardiac surgery children often show a cold, angry attitude toward their parents. We got none of that. Sierra was most eager to be with us. We detected no hostility and no withdrawal whatsoever. Of course, we attributed this healthy mood to our success at getting into the recovery room, as well as to her general excellent preparation. There was very little cause for Sierra to feel abandoned, tricked, surprised, angry, or any other terrible thing. She had known all that was going to happen, and it did. Furthermore, we were with her a third of the time in the recovery room, when she most needed us.

We brought some presents to her in the recovery room. In particular, a kite that someone had brought for her made a big impression. We had warned her that waking up in the recovery room would be hard, because she would have all these tubes in her, and would have strange nurses around, and lots of beepers going off from the machines, and that she would be extremely thirsty but nobody would give her anything to drink. Furthermore, her body might be all sore and achy. Knowing these things diminished the fear; it was OK, this was expected discomfort.

It wasn't so bad for her. Afterward she told John, "All those beepers sounded like birds chirping. And that was a nice kite."

Nonetheless, to us the moment they announced that she was coming up to the intensive care unit, where we could be with her every second without dodging head nurses, was the moment of delivery. Our hearts sang. She was coming. The worst was over. The surgery was complete. Our little girl was coming home to us. She was fully alive. The operation was a success. The suspense was over. Sierra was coming upstairs. Sierra was recovering: Sierra had made it. Sierra.

CHAPTER SEVENTEEN

The Intensive Care Unit

SIERRA LOOKED LIKE SHE'D been through the wringer. Her face was gray, her body limp and exhausted. Her eyelids drooped. Her hair was flattened down with sweat. Tubes extended from her nose, and there was no smile on her lips nor light in her eyes. Her sweet little self was as tired as it could be.

But she was conscious, and she was fixed. It wasn't long before she began to flicker back to herself. When I showed her a chocolate chip cookie, a Chunky, and a Reese Bar I had gotten for her, in a final abandonment of the earlier resolve not to yield to the desire to give her all the candy she wanted, her eyes shot open, probed John's and my smiling faces, and lit up. She was unchanged. A little candy could go a long way.

We sat by her. John sang and sang and sang, every song she had ever heard, and a lot of new ones too. She dozed and woke up. Every fifteen minutes her blood pressure cuff automatically started puffing up so her sleep was interrupted constantly.

We telephoned everyone. Happy phone calls buzzing through New York, and back and forth to Seattle, Boston,

San Francisco. We called Rodney, who was as jubilant as the closest members of our family.

Once the awesome wonder of it was absorbed, we began to attend to what Sierra seemed to need now, on a more subtle level. Since she was still busy saying, "No. Don't do it to me," to any approaching medical personnel, we decided to help her relieve and vent whatever feelings lay behind that. On the second day, we engaged one of the nurses to help us. We asked her to stand by the bed prior to taking Sierra's temperature and simply say, "I'm sorry, Sierra, I have to take your temperature."

We encouraged Sierra to go ahead and say, "NO! I don't want you to do it." Sierra said it with increasing force, over and over, while the nurse quietly repeated, "I have to do it." Sierra understood the game, and she burst out laughing, yelling, "NO! NO! NO! You can't do it!" Then she cried.

But in our judgment this little catharsis didn't finish the issue. She still seemed to us on the third day to be not just tired, but emotionally depressed. She was not hostile, but glazed over, down in the dumps, quiet, unresponsive. We felt she needed some emotional release of all the tension, as well as whatever she had experienced while unconscious in the operating room and while in the recovery room. The opportunity presented itself when it was time to take off the bandage. When the nurse told John this little ordeal was approaching, he arranged for the nurse not to just jerk it off, but to spend a long leisurely time with Sierra in the bathtub while John helped Sierra to release her feelings. Forty-five minutes they spent, with Sierra crying and yelling, sobbing and talking, while John nurtured her warmly and worked the bandage loose under the nurse's expert instructions.

When I found them later in the bed, Sierra was sparkling. Not just physically alive, she was now emotionally relieved and apparently happy. She was safely back in her parents' hands. And she had let fly a huge load of emotional distress.

From that moment on, we discerned no further depression, sadness, withdrawal, or even much tiredness. She was awake.

On the third morning. John was sitting next to Sierra's bed at dawn, quietly singing one of his favorite songs (By Laura Nyro) while Sierra dozed. He was in a deeply contemplative mood, relief and peacefulness having overcome him. The words of the song went like this:

> *And when I die*
> *And when I'm gone,*
> *There'll be one child born*
> *In this world*
> *To carry on,*
> *To carry on.*
> *There'll be one child born*
> *In this world*
> *To carry on,*
> *To carry on.*

A nurse called John to the phone. His mother said, "John, I'm sorry to call you at the hospital with this news, but your father just died."

CHAPTER EIGHTEEN

Life . . . and Death . . . Goes On

JOHN'S FATHER HAD BEEN seriously ill for some months. John and I both felt that his father had somehow found the strength to wait until he knew that his little granddaughter had survived the operation, and then he let himself pass away.

Meanwhile, Sierra recovered more rapidly than expected on the ward, and came happily home with John and me, clutching her bag of forty-three presents that she had received from members of the Sierra Stoneman-Bell Heart Club during her hospitalization. When we got home, we found a beautiful plant delivered by Rodney to mark the moment of continued healthy life. That plant continues to grow, thirty-nine years later, in our living room, despite the fact that Rodney himself passed away just a few years after Sierra's surgery. He had spent the last few years of his life intensifying his work as an advocate for parents.

Within a week of our return home from the hospital, I received a call from my mother: "Dorothy, your father has just had a severe heart attack. Please come home." This was unexpected, as my father had always seemed strong and healthy. Two months of medical and family drama with my father followed, culminating in his death in mid-August. His absence caused us to notice that my mother's mind had unraveled to a considerable extent. She was soon diagnosed as having Alzheimer's disease. This led inevitably to John, Sierra, and I moving to Massachusetts in 1985 to live with her and care for her until she passed away in 1987.

But these are all different stories, not to be told here.

Sierra flourished with no further symptoms or setbacks, and no apparent ill effects or even bad memories from her surgery. Certain memories stayed with her: among others, the boy with the stitches all over his head, the kite in the recovery room, the chocolate egg that she couldn't have and then she finally got, Megan's Wonder Woman underwear, and a basic good feeling about the whole thing.

We felt very deeply that as a family, supported by a community of friends and a collection of superb doctors and caring medical staff, we had absolutely done our best to ensure Sierra's well-being, on every level.

CHAPTER NINETEEN

Thirteen Years Later

Over the years I frequently pondered Dr. Doyle's warning. She had said, "Mrs. Stoneman, your letter says you do not want Sierra to be powerless in the hospital. If Sierra has power at age four, you'll be in trouble when she's 14."

Another respected colleague and friend had once said to me after observing my approach to teaching, "Dorothy, when you have children of your own, if you continue this attitude of trying to say "Yes" all the time, I pity the people who have to relate to your child."

At the time, I didn't believe either warning would turn out to be true, but I had sufficient doubt that I never forgot the remarks.

But if ever there was a danger, Sierra herself warded it off. At age eight, she said to me, "Mommy, you and Daddy have spoiled me. I want you to un-spoil me. If I always want my own way when I'm twenty, I don't think I'll have any friends." We agreed to say "No," more often to assist her campaign at self-improvement. We probably didn't change our ways for more than a month or so, but her request suggested to us that it is very difficult to spoil a child who feels well-loved and is learning positive values. Somehow the positive values were dominant.

In fact, Sierra's teenage years have been delightful, devoid of conflict with us, and free of any self-defeating behavior. Her life has been marked by an enormous degree of independent responsibility and high standards of achievement in every arena. She has grown into a young adult who invariably does her best at every challenge and displays a thoroughness coupled with a down-to-earth sense of right and wrong that will take her far in life. Her friendships have been deep and lasting.

In June of 1994, she graduated from Belmont Public High School as valedictorian. She was accepted on early admission into Brown University. She earned high awards in science, Spanish, English, basketball, track, orchestra, and student government. Her speech at graduation was an eloquent call for young people to take on the challenge of leadership in the world beyond their own personal lives. We couldn't have been more proud. She and her group of friends went on to make the news by renting a large school bus to attend the prom, prominently displaying a sign that said, "Drug free bus."

All the events surrounding her graduation seemed to mark the completion of our central role as her parents. She was definitely grown-up, and well launched. This moment of completion inspired me to finish this chronicle of her operation, which had lain in my desk drawer for twelve years, and finally prepare it for publication. It had always seemed that the usefulness of this document to other parents would depend not primarily on whether Sierra's operation was successful or not, because that was a product of the doctors' skill, but also on whether her development as a person revealed positive or negative effects of our approach to childrearing. If Dr. Doyle had been right, and Sierra developed into a wild hellion who made her parents suffer for years, I wouldn't be inviting people to read this book!

During the thirteen years between 1981 and 1994, we became increasingly convinced that although our cooperative, noncoercive approach led to some agonized moments of trial, it was essentially correct. Recently I have been in the position of counseling a family member who was facing a severe and debilitating emotional crisis, which he was convinced was rooted in a traumatic childhood experience of having been physically forced under anesthesia by his father, against the boy's most forceful protests, for a routine tonsillectomy. His continued anguish over the scars of this and related experiences made me grateful that we had not succumbed to the pressure to force Sierra into the operating room when the chips were down.

And now, at the moment we are actually moving to publish this story, in 2020, Sierra is the happy mother of her own beautiful son who is being raised with similar parenting approaches by her and her loving husband. No surgery is expected and all is well. We are all happy and healthy, grateful to be living such a full life!

Many thanks to the doctors and medical researchers who figured out how to save the lives of children like Sierra!

EPILOGUE

Reflections from Sierra, Thirty-nine Years Later

July 2020

READING THIS BOOK, YOU may wonder how I turned out, and whether my parents' approach to parenting through my heart surgery was successful, or ill-conceived . . . helpful or damaging? Here are a few reflections, thirty-nine years later, as I'm now parenting my own son who is about the same age I was during surgery.

My heart surgery was a traumatic life-threatening medical event, but my parents' approach and the support they had as they went through it with me minimized any lasting negative effects. The reality is that it was a very successful surgery that saved my life. I have lived most of my life like it never happened, as if I didn't have a serious congenital heart condition. I was an active child, I played competitive sports growing up, and didn't ever identify as having any physical weakness or defect.

As a young adult, after moving back to New York City, I had some chest pains and decided to seek out the same pediatric cardiology practice that guided me through my childhood surgery. I found wonderful, thoughtful doctors who had taken over for my previous cardiologist (it had been about twenty years). My heart was fine, but the doctor warned that if and when I decided to have my own children, I might have to plan for a caesarian birth because of the extra pressure childbirth could put on my repaired aorta. I was upset by this idea, but I took it in stride.

At thirty-nine, I gave birth to my first child under the coordinated care of my NYU cardiologist and OB/GYN doctors. I did end up having an emergency C-section, but not because of my heart condition. I had been cleared to push if I got that far, with close monitoring. After twenty-plus hours in labor, the baby's heart rate abruptly dropped, and the doctors decided they needed to get him out quickly. I was suddenly back on the operating table, feeling terrified but doing my best to stay connected to the little one about to be born. He arrived completely healthy and has been the light of my life ever since.

I still practice the same co-counseling process that my mom described in the book, because I found that it was helpful to me throughout my life. Through this practice, I have worked on feelings and memories that seem to stem from the surgery experience—some fear of dying, violent flashes that had related elements, fog from anesthesia. But I never lost my sense of myself, my connection to my parents, and the sense that they were looking out for me at every turn, that they would stand strong and advocate for what was best for me (even when it didn't fit with protocol—all the examples of saying "No"). I knew they were scared, but they stayed clear and confident and optimistic with me, while they got support from other adults to unload their fears and grief about the situation. As a result, their anxieties didn't land on me as I was trying to face this serious challenge with my life at stake. That was brilliant and powerful.

Amazingly, and probably as a result of the way my parents let me experience my feelings while going through the actual process, I have never had much residual conscious fear of doctors. I have had near fainting episodes in hospitals or in seeing scars, but nothing where I feel gripped with fear. I know other adults who had similar childhood surgeries and who are completely gripped by irrational fear in relation to medical treatment (and some other things).

I am part of the first generation of people born with this type of congenital heart defect who were able to have corrective surgery allowing us to live long full lives. At age forty-four, I have already lived twice as long as I likely would have without the surgery. At a recent visit with my cardiologist, who runs a clinic for adult patients with congenital heart conditions and who knows Dr. Doyle, my pediatric cardiologist, she mentioned that many adults with their own careers and families still come to their appointments with their parents because they don't fully understand their condition or treatment. She said my parents must have done a good job because of how I show up—I'm assuming she meant that I understand what I have, what happened, and how to take care of myself now. My parents always gave me information, even as a young child, so I knew what I would be facing and could understand it and be part of the decision-making, when possible. It is sometimes overwhelming to know what's coming, but I would rather know than be blindsided in the moment.

I am very grateful to my parents for their strength and smarts in shepherding me through the medical maze and for the life-saving medical care and technology that I had access to. I am still going strong, now raising my son with as much love and resilience as I got from my family. When I hear my mom's voice in this book, it reminds me how much parents love, how hard we work, and how vulnerable we feel as we move through the world with our children. It also shows how powerful it can be to stay close and stand up for our children through the challenges.

Made in the USA
Monee, IL
04 November 2026

67378962R00115